Property of:

Robert David Fink

3/1/67

D1297340

THE CHOICE OF
A MEDICAL CAREER

Essays on the Fields
of Medicine

THE CHOICE OF
A MEDICAL CAREER

Essays on the Fields of Medicine

Edited By

JOSEPH GARLAND, M.D., SC.D. (HON.)

Editor, *New England Journal of Medicine;*
Consultant Editor, British *Practitioner*

and

JOSEPH STOKES III, M.D.

Associate in Preventive Medicine,
Harvard Medical School;
Associate Editor, *New England Journal of Medicine*

SECOND EDITION

J. B. LIPPINCOTT COMPANY
Philadelphia • Montreal

Contributors

FRANCIS HEED ADLER, M.D.
Professor of Ophthalmology at the University of Pennsylvania

LEONA BAUMGARTNER, M.D.
Professor of Public Health and Preventive Medicine at Cornell University and Commissioner of Health, City of New York

WILLIAM B. BEAN, M.D.
Professor of Medicine and Head of the Department of Internal Medicine at the University of Iowa

C. SIDNEY BURWELL, M.D.
Samuel A. Levine Professor of Medicine Emeritus at Harvard Medical School

J. ENGLEBERT DUNPHY, M.D.
Professor of Surgery at the University of Oregon

JAMES E. ECKENHOFF, M.D.
Professor of Anesthesiology at the University of Pennsylvania and Editor of the Journal Anesthesiology

WILLIAM FEINDEL, M.D.
Professor of Neurosurgery at McGill University

HARRIET L. HARDY, M.D.
Assistant Medical Director and Chief of the Occupational Medical Service, Massachusetts Institute of Technology

J. HARTWELL HARRISON, M.D.
Clinical Professor of Genito-Urinary Surgery at Harvard Medical School

FRED JENNER HODGES, M.D.
Professor of Radiology at the University of Michigan

CHESTER M. JONES, M.D.
Clinical Professor of Medicine Emeritus at Harvard Medical School

CARROLL B. LARSON, M.D.
Professor of Orthopedic Surgery at the University of Iowa

FRANCIS L. LEDERER, M.D.
Professor of Otolaryngology at the University of Illinois

CLARENCE S. LIVINGOOD, M.D.
Director, Department of Dermatology at the Henry Ford Hospital, Detroit, Michigan; Editorial Board, A.M.A. Archives of Dermatology

H. HOUSTON MERRITT, M.D.
Professor of Neurology at Columbia University

DANIEL M. ROGERS, M.D.
Chairman, Publication Committee of American Academy of General Practice

JOHN ROMANO, M.D.
Professor of Psychiatry at the University of Rochester

ROBERT E. ROTHERMEL, M.D.
Director of Professional Education, New York City Department of Health

HOWARD A. RUSK, M.D.
Professor of Physical Medicine and Rehabilitation at New York University

JOSEPH STOKES, JR., M.D.
William H. Bennett Professor of Pediatrics, University of Pennsylvania

ROBERT E. STOWELL, M.D., PH.D.
Scientific Director, Armed Forces Institute of Pathology

BENJAMIN TENNEY, M.D.
Clinical Professor of Obstetrics and Gynecology at Harvard Medical School

LUTHER L. TERRY, M.D.
Surgeon General, U. S. Public Health Service

W. BARRY WOOD, JR., M.D.
Professor of Microbiology at Johns Hopkins University

Preface

Those of us who retain, however dimly, a picture of medical practice at the turn of the century must often marvel at the changes that it has undergone during these two generations. Medical practice was then almost entirely a matter of direct contact with the patient and of direct, usually unshared responsibility for his care. During this period much has been gained in the way of scientific progress; on the other hand, something in the way of kindly concern, of "caritas medici," as Dr. Bean terms it, although not lost, has tended to become less personal to many physicians and hardly enters into the daily life of too many others.

A profession that was once an art and to some extent a science has become an aggregate of various sciences, yet striving to remain to every possible degree an art. For if medicine is to continue with its primary function of service to the individual patient it must also continue to cultivate understanding and sympathetic communication with him. It must encourage this in the face of an increasing professional preoccupation with clinical specialization, practice by groups of physicians and surgeons, and the economic and political factors that threaten the traditional relation between doctor and patient.

Despite all the ramifications that medicine has undergone and the sweet uses of its diversity, most of which has been in the name of progress, one must still remember that the single purpose of the profession is the prevention of disease and the care of those who are ill. Such care is the direct function of the clinician, whether in the wards of an urban hospital or in the multiple responsibilities of a country practice. It is the indirect goal of the worker absorbed in the complicated tech- nics of a research laboratory, which has become a way of life for so many ardent investigators.

The total care of the patient, as Dr. Burwell suggests in his introductory chapter, is a happy blend of science and art, regardless of such categorical factors as specialties. He has also indicated the four cornerstones on which the structure of the profession rests: the care of the patient, teaching, re- search and administration.

This book consists of a series of original essays presenting the gradually acquired wisdom of a number of leaders in their respective fields. It is intended to convey to the student or the physician on the threshold of a medical career as complete a picture as possible of the profession to which he is dedicating himself and the opportunities that it presents. On a practical level it is intended to serve as a guide for the channeling of his life within that profession.

THE EDITORS.

Contents

THE CHOICE OF
A MEDICAL CAREER

Essays on the Fields
of Medicine

C. SIDNEY BURWELL, M.D.

Samuel A. Levine Professor of Medicine Emeritus at Harvard Medical School

1

The Art and the Science

An impressive characteristic of modern medicine is the rapidity of its change. Research in the biological sciences, the physical sciences, the medical sciences, and the phenomena of disease in patients has led to such changes that the medicine of today is quite different from the medicine of yesterday. Change continues at an increasing rate. These changes are in medicine itself and also in the social setting in which it serves.

The fact of change has implications for those who work in any part of the broad field of medicine. It is essential that such workers accept the responsibility of being continuous and life-long students. Their responsibility for continuing education never ends. The rapidity and the extent of changes in medicine also mean that individuals now in training for any of the diverse careers available in medicine must have a different kind of training from their predecessors. The fact that today's students must prepare themselves for tomorrow's medicine gives added importance to experience in the basic medical sciences since by and large the future changes in medicine will be understood best by those who are competent in these basic sciences.

Another impressive characteristic of current medicine is the degree of specialization that has developed. It is often said that knowledge has grown to such a degree that it is no longer possible for one mind to achieve expertness in all its fields. Since expert knowledge and expert skill are required for the optimum care of patients and for the further advance of

knowledge, the principle of specialization has been a necessary one. It is, however, not without disadvantages and hazards. One danger, particularly evident in the narrower and
more technical specialties, is that their practitioners, though
highly skilled in the science and technology of the special
field, may lose sight of the total problems and their relation
to it. This danger is reduced, though certainly not eliminated,
by two factors. The first of these is the common experience
that all doctors have had in taking the courses leading to the
M.D. degree, and the happy circumstance that wise men continue their general education in medicine as well as their
special training. A second influence, effective in the case of
physicians involved in the care of individual patients, is the
biological fact that the unit of medical care is an indivisible
patient.

One of the results of the phenomenon of specialization has
been a broadening of the spectrum of opportunity confront-
ing the medical graduate. A doctor's life is a series of decisions
affecting his career. At some time in their lives men and
women make the original decision to enter the broad field of
medicine. When they have attained the M.D. degree new
decisions must be made regarding the area in which further
training is to be sought and in which their professional life
is to be lived. It is with the types of work and opportunity and
the varieties of preparation for them that this book will in
general be concerned.

Subsequent chapters of this volume will describe a wide
and interesting variety of careers distinguished from one another mainly by the subject matter and the methods of one
field as compared with others. Before you turn to these discussions of differences, let us consider certain characteristics
of all medical careers.

In general, the activities of doctors may be conveniently
described in four categories:

1. The care of patients
2. Teaching
3. Research
4. Administration

Most doctors do all of these things, but different doctors do them in widely varying proportion. For example, those who enter careers in the medical sciences will participate in teaching, in research, and in administration, but will usually not be directly involved in the care of patients. Those who spend essentially full time in the practice of medicine will devote most of their time to the care of patients, some time in administrative activities connected with the organization of that care, and most of them will do some teaching. Let us, however, consider briefly each of these four subdivisions of activity.

The Care of Patients. The care of the sick is traditionally the duty of physicians. Supplying guidance and help to individual patients is to many doctors a remarkably satisfying combination of science and art. The opportunities and satisfactions of this unusual combination have been described eloquently and clearly by Atchley in an illuminating article entitled, "The Healer and the Scientist." Both science and art are indispensable in the best care of patients; they are not incompatible with one another, but complementary. Many of the careers to be considered in subsequent chapters are varieties of practice. Some of these varieties, for example internal medicine, are wide fields, so wide that their practitioners should perhaps be referred to as "generalists." Other varieties are more restricted. They may be restricted to a special organ, as in the case of ophthalmology, or to a method of procedure, as in the case of radiology. A man making a decision among the various varieties of practice will take account of his interest in the subject matter, and will reflect on the kind of responsibility he wishes to assume, and will consider his particular talents, and the opportunities that present themselves or that can be found. He will also consider whether he prefers working as a member of a team or as an independent or lone worker. Neither method is out of date, and some people fit one category better than the other.

The care and treatment of sick people is not all there is to patient care. Another aspect of the care of patients has become of increasing significance in every field of medicine. This is the area of the maintenance of health and the prevention of disease. This is part of the duty of everyone who takes care of individual patients and has also developed into a highly important special field in which the unit of practice is groups of people rather than individuals.

Preparation for a career in any field devoted mainly to practice should be planned in the light of an important recent development in medicine. The major contribution of the twentieth century to medicine is increasing knowledge of the physiology of disease and the management of disease in the light of this increasing knowledge. Therefore, the preparation for the care of patients should give special emphasis to the understanding of disease in terms of physiology.

Teaching. Teaching is as much a traditional obligation of doctors as is the care of the sick, particularly as it applies to the instruction of the next generation of physicians. Teaching also offers durable satisfactions, particularly the satisfaction of seeing students develop into effective and independent individuals. Teaching as a part of careers in medicine is of almost infinite variety. It may, in the case of an individual physician, involve candidates for the M.D. degree, candidates for the Ph.D. in one of the basic sciences, training in one of the special fields in which medicine is divided, the training of auxiliary personnel, the organization of opportunities for keeping up with the prodigious advances in medicine, and many other varieties. Teaching in medicine is at its best when it does not exist by itself, but when it is carried on in combination with the care of patients, or with research, or with both. Teaching, research, and the care of patients strengthen and supplement each other, and the joint enterprise helps avoid one of the major dangers to individual careers in medicine—namely, failing to keep up with the incredibly rapid changes.

Research. Research is for some people an essential form of activity and such individuals will be productive of new knowledge even under conditions of limited opportunity. For others, research is non-essential, and many of these are admirable physicians and excellent teachers. Fields of research are

almost limitless, and in this area there is probably more indi-
vidualization of careers than in any other general sphere of
activity.

Doctors of medicine may investigate the phenomena and
mechanisms of disease, and by so doing improve the science
and the art of medicine. Studies of the phenomena of disease
in patients can also contribute importantly to the basic medical sciences. One should not make the mistake of thinking
that so-called clinical research ("clinical" here is used purely
in the sense of relating to patients) is necessarily directed to
practical and immediate ends. Many fascinating chapters in
the knowledge of the basic medical sciences—for example, the
physiology and biochemistry of the endocrine glands—have
been initiated and advanced by the perceptive observation
and study of patients. Of course, systematic studies in patients
are often directed to the improvement of methods of diagnosis and treatment, but the more basic part of clinical investigation has to do with the exploration of the great series of
biological experiments performed by disease. These experiments of nature can be studied and can add to our knowledge
of both biology and medicine.

The opportunities for research open to the man with an
M.D. degree are as wide as his imagination. He may work in
theoretical physics, in the chemistry of the cellular nucleus,
in sociology, or in the relief of itching. In my opinion most
research in the basic medical sciences and in the study of the
phenomena of disease should be done in association with universities by people who participate in the teaching of students at various stages of their experience. It has already been
said that participation in research is good for teaching. It is
for most people equally true that responsibility for teaching
is good for their research.

Administration. It is fashionable to criticize the necessity
for administrative activity on the part of scientists, and it is
true that some individuals have permitted their administrative duties to devour them. It is also true that some
organizations have permitted administrative duties to inter-

rupt promising research and teaching careers. However, there are important and absorbing careers in administration. For people whose talents and interests are in this direction there are great opportunities for productive service contributing to research, to teaching, and to the care of patients. Examples are to be found in such fields as preventive medicine, public health, hospital administration, and education. Most of these careers will be full-time careers in administration, and to have able, devoted, and knowledgeable people in high administrative posts is essential if medicine is to serve the community well. Some careers in administration require a person who has had medical training; some do not.

It should also be said that administration is part of the job of everybody in medicine, and one of the responsibilities that should be assumed by those who provide training opportunities for young people in medicine is responsibility for some basic instruction in principles of administration. Poor administration interferes with the care of patients, with teaching, and with research. Good administration is a help to all and serves to free professional personnel for professional activities. Experience would seem to indicate that the most important quality of good administration is clarity, especially clarity in the location of responsibility.

* * * *

The rapidity of change in medicine, which has been emphasized, means that types of careers in medicine will also change. Therefore, do not think that the careers available to you are limited to the varieties you see around you among your senior colleagues. New and interesting careers will be developed in this generation as they have been in earlier generations, and people entering medicine today will be the ones who develop them. It is true that certifying boards, and increasing departmentalization of medical schools and hospitals, suggest a crystallization of the types of careers, but one should not be misled by the apparent rigidity of these patterns. The patterns are not really fixed. Subject matter in each department is changing, and the relation of one department to another is changing. This is not always apparent to a superficial view. Let me cite an example. If one compares the general outline of the curriculum in a medical school catalogue of 1900 with the general outline of the curriculum in a catalogue of 1950, he will often be struck by their similarity, although he knows that the content of the curriculum is deeply and radically altered. Many curricular plans are a little like the shelves in a pharmacy. The bottles are still the same shape, but the contents are different.

A concept of continuing change is essential in planning training programs leading to various types of careers. It appears that individuals entering various careers today should not be trained as were the people who are now leaders in those fields. They should be trained for some approximation of what the special field may be twenty-five years from now. This suggests that the people who plan the education of young men in medicine should be the young men themselves. They can be helped by advice; they can be helped by the opportunity of systematic experience, but they must have the opportunity to use their own imaginations to try to think ahead and to make their own plans. The most interesting careers are those that are created by originality and foresight. Some of these will be created within the existing framework. Others will be additions or replacements.

Some of the changes in medicine will be due to advancing knowledge in the sciences basic to medicine. Some will be due to advancing knowledge of the mechanisms of disease. Some will be due to changes in the incidence and even in the nature of disease processes as man changes his environment. Some will be due to alterations in the social setting in which medicine plays its role.

Happily, there are some things about medicine that do not change. One of these is the nature of the relevant organism—namely, man. Another is the nature of the responsible relation between doctor and patient. Finally, there is another characteristic of medicine that does not change—that is, that in any career in this general field there is the possibility of a happy, productive, and useful life. Careers in medicine differ in the kind of problem they present and in the kind of talents they require, but they do not differ in nobility. It is as good to do one kind of medicine as another; it is as good to take care of patients as to teach; it is as good to teach as to do research; it is as good to do research as to take care of patients.

All types of careers in medicine offer opportunity for usefulness, accomplishment, originality, scholarship, and magnanimity. Thus careers in medicine can lead to solid and durable satisfactions. There is, however, no evidence that these solid and durable satisfactions are available to anyone unless he earns them.

REFERENCE

Atchley, Dana W.: The Healer and the Scientist. The Saturday Review, January 9, 1954.

Daniel M. Rogers, M.D.

Chairman, Publication Committee of American Academy of General Practice

2

General Practice

Unlike students in other disciplines leading to the doctorate degree, medical students constitute a fairly homogeneous body participating in approximately the same courses until graduation. Exceptionally, prior training or the inspiration received in an elective course leads the student, while still an undergraduate, to select a special interest for further development after graduation from medical school. In general, however, the choice of the type of medical practice is not fixed until the end of the senior year or during the first year of hospital internship. Since the nature of further training will depend on the type of practice, this is the time for decision. Serious consideration should be given to general practice, which can offer the greatest challenge and a bountiful life to one with the proper attributes and training.

Stripped of the implications of military organization, such as rank and regimentation, the position of general staff officer corresponds to a degree to that of a general practitioner; the term "general" has much the same connotation. The aspirant to general practice needs not only a broad training in the total field of medicine from a practical as well as a theoretical standpoint; he must also have intrinsically the philosophic outlook that can grasp a broad subject properly to correlate its component parts. He must be conversant to an appropriate degree with all the major branches of medicine—internal medicine, surgery, obstetrics, pediatrics, public health, and the rest, for he will be called upon to exercise his talents in diverse fields day after day. One of the attractions of general practice is its variety.

Commonly the general practitioner is the first to see the patient regardless of the complaint or the ultimate disposition of the case. It is his responsibility to evaluate the situation: Will the services of a specialist be required? Should the patient be hospitalized or can he handle the case adequately in the home or office—perhaps with the aid of laboratory data and the visiting nurse?

These questions make it apparent that the first requirement in general practice is keen diagnostic acumen. Laboratory aids are of value in confirming a diagnosis, but on many occasions the general physician is confronted with problems he must meet with his own resources exclusively, *sans* hospitals, *sans* consultants. The second requirement, then, is that he must be self-reliant.

Self-reliance must not be confused with over-confidence; no general practitioner is equally qualified in all fields. Although nationwide statistics show that the well-trained general physician can handle 80 per cent of all the problems he sees, he must be the first to recognize his personal limitations, consulting with a specialist or referring the patient to one. His special interest will lead him to emphasize one branch of medicine in his training; in his chosen field he may approximate the capability of the specialist.

Published studies of the composition of general practices indicate that the bulk of the cases fall into the category of upper respiratory or cardiorespiratory diseases, but this is somewhat misleading. A corresponding practice analysis by a group of three internists produced a very similar result. The significance is merely that the general practices analyzed happened to be more heavily inclined toward internal medicine. In some areas of the country, however, most of the simpler major surgery is capably performed by general practitioners; many are highly trained in obstetrics, anesthesiology, or psychiatry; some have made a secondary career of public health.

The agnomen most cherished by the general practitioner seems to be "family physician." The image of the family physician today is a far cry from the connotation of several decades ago that evoked the concept of a sincere but overworked doctor with a limited background of education and training. The training for general practice is little different except in content from that for certain specialty practices. The distinction in practice is that the general physician is well equipped to minister to the medical needs of the entire family, treating the individuals composing it as a group in relation to their native environment. This maintains a proper sociologic and psychological relation conducive to intra- and inter-personal harmony. The basic importance of the relation of environment to disease has been acknowledged by a change in undergraduate teaching in some medical schools. Western Reserve University pioneered in this departure several years ago by assigning a selected family to the entering student as his "patients" to follow throughout the four years. A similar experiment is in progress in the Department of Pediatrics at Harvard. The students taking their clinical work in pediatrics at the Massachusetts General Hospital make house calls and a family study of cases assigned to them from those they see in the outpatient department. The student is encouraged not only to consult with the visiting and resident pediatric staff, but also to pursue as far as need be the social and medical affairs of the rest of the family at home and in other departments of the hospital.

The family physician assumes an implicit responsibility for total family care. Although he may share his responsibility with a specialist who renders definitive service on specific occasions, he will advise the family on which specialist to select and hence is ultimately responsible to his patients because of his choice of consultants. The family will turn to its family physician for guidance in all medical (and many nonmedical) affairs—they will also come to him for explanation or progress reports whenever one of their number is under a specialist's care.

Frequently the family physician will collaborate with the

specialist in the care of a sickness or injury. The former will commonly be called in consultation by his specialist colleague, for the patient whom he has referred, to supply background data or advise on a course of action that his intimate knowledge of the patient as a social organism can most readily provide.

The thesis has occasionally been advanced that general practice is a decadent branch of medicine ultimately to disappear. It will be replaced, it is suggested, by a complex medical group consisting of a corps of medical specialists and ancillary personnel specializing in various paramedical fields such as sociology, psychology, and the like.

Two serious defects of such a scheme are immediately manifest: such a project can scarcely be supported by the economics of practice, except in a large metropolitan area, without recourse to socialized medicine. Furthermore, what happens to the unfortunate patient or the corresponding sociological unit, the family, when he or it becomes so fractionated? The strong allegiance that the family develops for its medical counselor would be diluted to the point of dissipation.

It is apparent that conscientious fulfillment of the role of general physician involves participation in community life for a better understanding of the patient's environment; in the smaller communities the physician works and often relaxes with his patients—without losing the dignity of his professional relation. The community, furthermore, because of this very relation expects the family physician to be a leader in molding its affairs.

It has traditionally been the peculiar privilege of the family physician to occupy a position of esteem with his patients; but what of his relation to other physicians? Here he has lost ground as specialization took over. Scarcely more than a decade ago scant attention was paid by educators to formal postgraduate training for general practitioners. And they were, on the whole, a pretty motley group—some were distinguished physicians, many were looked upon as the hacks of the profession, content to be the yeomen of the guard, while the specialists manned the loftier ramparts of medical science. Only the latter enjoyed the privilege of a training designed to equip them for a specific field of practice.

A change was wrought when a small group of distinguished general practitioners, dedicated to their field as a cause to be espoused, organized the American Academy of General Practice. The Academy brought general practice into sharper focus as a specialized branch of medicine; it has been highly instrumental in initiating formalized postgraduate training for this field. By establishing a high standard of performance for membership and requiring continuing study by its members, it has forged a standard for general practice on a par with that of the specialties.

The following excerpts from the by-laws of the Academy of General Practice define acceptable training for the general practitioner:

> "Eligibility: To be eligible for active membership he must be of high moral and professional character. He must have been graduated from a medical school approved by the American Medical Association. He must be duly licensed to practice . . . and must be a member of . . . the American Medical Association or Canadian Medical Association . . . Candidates . . . must have had at least one year of rotating internship [at an approved hospital]. In addition he must have completed one of the following: (1) Two years of graduate training acceptable to and approved by the Commission on Education or (2) one year of graduate training . . . followed by two years of general practice."

> (Those graduating from medical school prior to January 1, 1966 may substitute three years of general practice for the latter requirement.)

One example of the recognition now accorded to this estate is the increasing development in hospitals of departments of general practice ranking equally with medicine, surgery, and the like. There was a tendency in the medically sheltered populous communities for the specialists to assume that the hospital was their exclusive domain. The reversal of this trend has been due largely to the influence of the Academy of General Practice. The Academy has promulgated the principle that hospital privileges should be granted to all practitioners commensurate to their ability as judged by an appropriate standard. Admission of general practitioners to hospital staffs in some areas is contingent upon membership in the Academy. Such membership should be the aim of every general practitioner. It constitutes his hallmark.

Many general practitioners are content to make a career simply of being good family physicians; but an increasing proportion find the stimulus of accomplishment leads them to seek further goals in the medical sphere for which their broad training and experience have adapted them. When accompanied by appropriate personality attributes they are peculiarly fitted for positions of responsibility in administrative fields. The military services have repeatedly stressed the importance of general training for a career in the medical corps. A significant number of outstanding general practitioners who received national attention, often through their work in medical organizations, are serving in a consultant capacity to the Air Force, Army, and Navy, or with branches of the National Institutes of Health.

In like manner general physicians have found their training valuable for posts as hospital administrators and in industrial medicine, insurance, public health, medical journalism, and, of course, teaching.

An increasing number of medical schools, recognizing that general practice is becoming more clearly defined as a special branch of medicine, are establishing departments of general practice. The clinical teaching involved is rendered intramurally in large degree by general practitioners, and extramurally, in some schools, by preceptorships.

No greater challenge exists for the young man studying medicine than general practice. The qualities of leadership, the breadth of interest, an insatiable thirst for knowledge, versatility, and love of one's fellows are basic requisites. He is a captain who roams the seven seas of medicine, at home in any port, but ready to call upon the specialist for guidance or special care in any situation surpassing his competence. He is the executive, however, who directs the medical team in the care of the family unit, who arrays the battery of pertinent laboratory studies, who summons the community's resources to supplement his personal care.

General practice knows no geographic bounds; it is needed on the high seas, in the cities and the suburbs and in the remote areas of the earth. The individual physician may decide where he would like to live and work. If the family practice of medicine is not enough to satisfy him, a vista of larger responsibilities beckons from his expanding horizon.

CHESTER M. JONES, M.D.

*Clinical Professor of Medicine Emeritus at
Harvard Medical School*

3

Internal Medicine

Any precise definition of the practice of internal medicine, or of an internist, is quite obviously impossible. Rather, it is important to describe the current significance of these terms by outlining the steps needed to prepare a physician for such a professional career and to discuss the opportunities and the responsibilities that are an integral part of such a career.

The practice of internal medicine, as a specialty, demands first an arduous and thorough training under critical supervision. In general, the internist is trained to diagnose and treat medically the "internal diseases" that afflict the adult. As a base, his practice embraces general and adequate knowledge of several specialties, although obviously the internist cannot know all the rapidly expanding details that enter into all special fields of medicine. Nevertheless, his training must provide him with the knowledge of how to recognize disease of one or another of the systems of the body and where to look for detailed information to guide him in diagnosis and intelligent therapy. At the same time, he must be able to recognize special gaps in his own knowledge and to admit them. The competent internist must have learned the hard discipline of saying, "I don't know," with the immediate addition of the words, "but I will find out."

The training that will provide the essentials must, if possible, be obtained in an institution where there is a tradition

16

of thoroughness and inquiry. The training center must set and demand high standards of adequacy, and supervision must be critical, albeit not unfriendly. A sense of personal responsibility must be an integral part of such training, regardless of the expenditure of time and effort. Therefore, this training must start with an internship in a hospital where such a tradition is nurtured and where house staff and active staff membership embody these qualities. During internship and subsequent training, the attainment of clinical maturity and the acquisition of newer scientific knowledge must be recognized as the essentials of a good training in internal medicine. To provide for this there must be adequate modern facilities and a clear designation of responsibility for excellent patient care, with critical supervision of younger men by older, experienced clinicians and teachers.

An internship in such an institution provides essentially an opportunity for learning proper habits of inquiry and patient care, which in turn lead to the development of a discipline of professional behavior that will last through professional life. Further resident training should follow, with its added opportunity for clinical and scientific experiences that lead continuously toward the professional maturity that is essential to a good internist. During these early years there should constantly be the urge to progress further in the understanding of the whys and the wherefores of mechanisms that underlie symptoms and the manifestations of disease. The atmosphere in which younger men work must be one in which there is no sharp distinction between "scientific" and "practical" medicine. Whatever is truly scientific is undoubtedly practical when it is understood and is integrated into that complex equation that we call "a sick patient." The scientific use and the practical use of newer knowledge are in no way mutually exclusive, and the integration of the two is not only essential but provides real protection against the dangers of superficial routines and more or less empirical decisions and therapeutic measures. The training, then, is long and arduous, but it lays the foundation for professional acumen and careful thought.

Although training in research is not a *sine qua non* of the training of an internist, the opportunity for developing investigative skills warrants a comment. Such an opportunity under good auspices provides a young physician with a special discipline—that of self-criticism. Meticulous attention to minute details, careful observations and equally careful conclusions, all subject to close scrutiny, provide a young man with a much more thoughtful attitude toward future problems than may otherwise obtain, and move the potential internist one step further toward his goal of clinical maturity.

The intern and residency years, with or without some experience in medical research, will usually cover a period of four to five years. In general, these years should include sufficient exposure to patient care to ensure a broad base of continuing clinical experience. Several avenues then are apparent for future development. Some special field in medicine may provide a source for further study and for the development of a particular proficiency and interest. Too early attention to subspecialties is rarely desirable, with the possible exception of those brilliant few individuals who will work in basic research. These latter may well add greatly to our knowledge of medical science, but more frequently than not they do not qualify as internists but rather as contributors to newer knowledge of fundamental principles. On the other hand, many internists may use the broad base of a good training in internal medicine to acquire special skill in the handling of patients with specific problems, such as those relating to cardiovascular or pulmonary disorders, digestive tract disease, and the like, and may become extremely valuable as special consultants. However, there are few diseases that can be included in the list of medical disorders that do not involve, during their course, abnormalities in the functioning of more than one body system—a fact that continually emphasizes the importance of a broad base of training and clinical experience, if proper judgments and decisions are to be maintained.

A further opportunity that may be available to the internist is that of teaching, the importance of which cannot be over-emphasized. From the time of Hippocrates the responsibility of older, experienced men to instruct and aid younger physicians has been accepted tacitly or openly. What has not been so generally accepted is the fact that a serious attempt to teach, whether it be in an academic milieu or in a non-university setting, benefits the teacher as much as the taught. The younger physicians of today are, for the most part, the recipients of a rapidly expanding fund of medical knowledge. Mutual discussion of problems by experienced clinicians and younger men in training is always a two-way road. Such discussions always lead to greater knowledge and a greater clarity of thought concerning bedside problems. The older physician, even if he be but slightly older, not only fulfills part of his obligations to the profession, and indirectly to the community, by devoting some time to teaching, but he also gains in understanding. This is particularly true of physicians who are trained as internists, inasmuch as it provides for a continuation of self-education that is essential to complete clinical maturity and for a continuing growth in professional stature.

It will be obvious that a sacrifice of time and energy must be compounded into the elements of a good internist, in order to reap the ultimate rewards. As Osler pointed out, the life of an internist is divided into three periods: "ten years for bread, ten years for bread and butter, and twenty years for cakes and ale." However, the satisfaction and the enthusiasm that can be derived from such an experience is enormous. With good training as a base and with continued experience, confidence emerges that fully justifies the expectation that an internist may arrive at the position of a respected consultant. Any well-matured internist has a right to expect this, with its rewards of professional recognition and patient satisfaction. However, certain attitudes and practices must be observed before such recognition is deserved and granted. An internist must be competent and at the same time aware of the advantages that he has gained or has been granted in early training opportunities. Humility, but not self-deprecation, is still a virtue, if for no other reason than the fact that no one is omniscient. Professional chauvinism must be studiously avoided, and the intelligent internist must recognize worth in other physicians and other institutions than his own. Medicine must still be a profession and not a trade. Adequate financial recompense for care and thoughtful consideration of a patient's problems is a reasonable expectation, but a primary interest in the making of money and the desire to drive a Cadillac instead of a Ford have wrecked for many a well-trained physician the respect that is due from his colleagues and his community.

A final comment is needed today regarding the relations between a competent internist and his patients. With the rapid and at times amazing advances in medical knowledge and scientific technics, and with the added fact that a steadily increasing number of patients are being cared for in hospitals, there is a mounting tendency to concentrate on the problem, rather than on the patient and his problems. This impersonal approach at times defeats the purpose of good medicine. Scientific knowledge is essential to adequate and effective therapy. However, as Peabody so aptly phrased it in his classic treatise, *The Care of the Patient,* "the treatment of disease may be entirely impersonal; the care of the patient must be completely personal." Without question, the understanding of a patient can be a science, which takes training, time and great experience. It also requires an interest, which cannot be feigned. The internist must be the person to whom the patient turns for final decisions, for adequate explanations and for the confidence that he inspires. A well-trained internist with a broad basic training will have learned the discipline of a careful history, an excellent and thorough physical examination, and a thoughtful choice of indicated laboratory studies that are the basis of good medical practice. The substitution of a multiplicity of routine procedures and short, superficial visits with the patient will not provide the basis for critical judgments and satisfactory results. Once the discipline is learned and experience gained, there need be no fear of inadequate professional recognition or insufficient monetary reward.

In summary, the terms "internist" and "internal medicine" imply long and careful training, leading to the acquisition of knowledge and the disciplines involved in its use. The training base must be initially broad but may well include added experience in some special smaller field of medicine. In order to continue to learn, an internist should engage in some form of teaching. At the same time, he must attempt to familiarize himself with current medical literature and should attend and actively participate in meetings where scientific and clinical subjects are discussed. Finally, he must accept the responsibility of patient care, as well as the care of disease, with the added obligation of recognizing the frequent necessity of obtaining help from others with special skills, without relinquishing his interest and concern in his patient. Only by combining these habits and qualities will his position as one trained in internal medicine be recognized by the public whom he serves. The need for such trained physicians is steadily increasing, and the ultimate opportunities for such professional maturity are endless.

REFERENCES

Osler, William: Aequanimitas, Internal Medicine as a Vocation, H. K. Lewis, London, 1904, p. 139.

Peabody, Francis Weld, M.D.: The Care of the Patient, J.A.M.A. *88*:877, 1927.

JOSEPH STOKES, JR., M.D.
William H. Bennett Professor of Pediatrics,
University of Pennsylvania

4

Pediatrics

Man's "nature is subdued to what it works in." The significant line of Shakespeare's is especially applicable to those whose lives are spent in the care, the nurture and the understanding of infants, children and adolescents. Today, the pediatrician, the general practitioner, the child psychiatrist and to some extent those in preventive medicine and public health are all joining together to support the family through the apprenticeship to life of their children. The gentle insight of the wise teacher, the experienced support of the family physician beloved by children, the perceptive touch of a grandmother in her preservation of the continuity of the cultural heritage, all eloquently attest to the profound influence that children and youth may have upon those who rightly and maturely serve them.

Pediatrics is sometimes considered as internal medicine covering a special age range from the neonatal period through adolescence. But it is more than this; it is not the age range primarily that sets it apart from internal medicine, but rather that it deals with the growing organism from the embryo to adult life with all the unique physical, psychological and social problems that bear directly on such growth and development. Thus by growth and development the parameters of normality common to both child and adult in a host of homeostatic regulatory mechanisms assume entirely new dimensions

22

in the child. Immunology, nutrition, metabolism, salt and fluid balance and endocrinology and all of the specialities of medicine have a host of variables affecting the premature infant, the newborn, the child and the adolescent—all quite different from those in the adult. Such variables also exist for each of these periods of growth in the psychological and social areas—all bearing on the physical health.

Pediatrics also is distinct from all other areas of medicine in two respects: the joy derived from the hopefulness inherent in the care of the young and the fact that it deals with medical problems in their purest form before complicating factors have obscured the basic elements of health and disease.

Pediatrics has kept pace with the major trend in all the biologic sciences—namely, to explore life in its natural biologic sequences from the single cell to the multicellular organism, from the embryo to the fully grown adult, and from the young to the adolescent. It is in these vital sequences and in the opportunity to influence and support them that pediatrics serves its major purpose. It is still a young and rapidly growing specialty and beckons the young in spirit to grow with it and to develop it further. The panorama of medicine covered by my own father in 60 years of general practice, beginning in 1883, points up the drama of an era of progress. As an intern he operated with D. Hayes Agnew, professor of surgery at the University of Pennsylvania, who in abdominal operations always turned up his boot, sharpened his knife on it and then proceeded to open the abdomen. Compare this with my father's experience over 60 years later of watching patients responding to penicillin. During the period of his lifetime the biologic sciences through Pasteur's work had reverted to the study of the growth and development of the bacterial cell and through Virchow's work had started exploring the growth and development of the animal cell and its relation to the whole organism. As the new experimental and technical methods of biochemistry, physiology and biophysics brought biologic and medical sciences back to the natural sequence of proceeding from the study of the unicellular to the multicellular organism, anatomy, pathology, microbiology, and pharmacology all joined in this universal effort.

I have sketched this pattern because it is essential to realize that the natural biologic sequence of development of knowledge in the clinical field from prenatal to adult life has also been reversed in medical teaching. Thus the sequence of subjects in medical teaching usually recapitulated their historical development at least in the relative emphasis accorded them. In the recent study conducted by Dr. Robert Aldrich, chairman of the Educational Committee of the American Pediatric Society, more than a 5th of the practicing pediatricians in the United States responded to his queries. They were asked to list in order of importance the 37 subjects that they had been taught in medical school. Anatomy was rated 1st in terms of training content and 18th in importance to them in their practice, whereas surgery was 7th in the amount of training and 35th in importance. By contrast is the fact that psychological problems were accorded 31st place in teaching content but 7th place in importance in actual practice. Thus the historically older subjects of anatomy and surgery tended to limit the students' opportunities to obtain newer knowledge increasingly needed.

During the 19th century sick infants and children were mistreated in general hospitals. Instances were recorded where 6 to 8 ill children were often packed into the same bed or placed in beds occupied by desperately ill adults. For such reasons the first children's hospital was founded in Paris in 1802, and the first in the English-speaking world in London in 1852—The Hospital for Sick Childen in Great Ormond Street. These were joined shortly by the first children's hospital in the Western Hemisphere, in Philadelphia, which opened its doors in 1855. Charles Dickens' impassioned plea,[1] at the Great Ormond Street Hospital soon after its founding, for the care of desperately ill and neglected infants and children is a stirring indictment of this "social cancer" and should be read by everyone interested in the history and the progress of medicine. Just as had been true in prison reform and in the development of nursing, women often led the way as they showed basic affection and understanding of young children.

Also historically, the lag of interest in, and development of, pediatrics resulted from the fact that it is more difficult to communicate directly with a patient than in most other specialties. There are also problems in applying to small infants and children methods and technics developed for adults. The urine sample, the spinal fluid and even the specimen of blood all require special patience and technic.

Medical students, like most young men and women, usually develop interest in infants and children only after they marry and have children of their own. Also, as individuals mature, they tend to develop interest in such fields as preventive medicine and public health, which are so closely related to pediatrics and general practice. In an interesting study[2] conducted by Dr. Helen H. Gee, Director of Research for the Association of American Medical Colleges, the Allport-Vernon-Lindzey Scale of Values was applied to both college and medical students from all sections of the United States. The Scale of Values includes the Theoretical, Economic, Aesthetic, Social, Political and Religious indices which cannot be fully clarified here. However, she says "the Social Value which the A-V-L authors describe as valuing the altruistic and philanthropic aspects of love of mankind is markedly lacking among the characteristics of most medical students." The Social value in fact is the lowest one of the 6 named above among medical students. Undergraduate college students studied in a similar manner with the same tests score much higher on the Social value. That such an outlook may militate against an interest in infants and children is problematic. It is apparent that as women have entered medicine the interest in the care of infants and children has deepened, although the significance of this has not been fully determined. It is also of interest that those students in this study who entered pediatrics as a specialty obtained higher Social value scores than all other career-choice groups except psychiatrists.

MAJOR HISTORICAL TRENDS

The major steps in the development of pediatrics and pediatric hospitals from the 19th century to the present were briefly as follows:

The general revulsion against the serious neglect of infants and children in general hospitals, resulting in the founding of children's hospitals.

The isolation in the latter part of the 19th century of infants and children with certain acute communicable diseases (e.g., scarlet fever, measles, and so forth) in separate "pest houses" or so-called "contagious" hospitals.

The placing in the early 20th century of newborn, premature and very young infants in the care of pediatricians and the orienting of their care toward pediatric hospitals.

The organization in medical schools of departments of pediatrics, first under, and finally separate from, departments of medicine. The development of full-time clinical chairs of pediatrics was the latest and most important part of this change. (See Academic Pediatrics below.)

The development of pediatric clinics for the prevention of disease and for the promotion and the teaching of child health, usually in close proximity or relation to pediatric hospitals and departments of pediatrics.

The awareness by surgeons in more recent years of the special problems presented by children and infants, especially in the field of congenital anomalies, and the development of "full-time" skilled pediatric surgeons for pediatric hospitals.

The rapid decline in recent years in severe infectious diseases, as a result of sulfonamides and antibiotics, which has completely changed the complexion of pediatric admissions to hospitals.

The growing awareness of the importance of the psychological development of the infant and the child in his family, his school and in his entire social milieu, with the resultant development in association with children's hospitals of child guidance clinics, social case work, leisure-time activities in hospitals and parent education.

The decreasing necessity for entire concentration on the saving of life and the increasing awareness of the need for improving the satisfactions in living for psychologically and physically handicapped infants and children, with resultant development of clinics in children's hospitals for such insults to, or defects of, the central nervous system as cerebral palsy, retardation, epileptiform seizures, autism or other severe psychological problems or neuromuscular diseases.

The natural interest of pediatricians and others in growth and development, reaching over into the seriously neglected adolescent area.

The continuously narrowing gap between the interests and the work of departments of medicine and pediatrics, between general hospitals and children's hospitals, and between the care of children and of adults in public health centers associated with medical schools, and a growing understanding of the frequent need for handling the family as a unit in health and disease, as well as the need for the co-ordinated long-term study of health and disease which reaches into every medical field from the beginning to the end of life.

The rapidly increasing availability of good pediatric care in suburban and outlying hospitals by the highly qualified pediatricians who are being trained in children's hospitals and are moving to such communities in large numbers.

The increasing understanding of the need for intensification of research and the provision of facilities in which to conduct it.

THE PROJECTION OF FUTURE TRENDS

The preceding review of major historical trends reveals the existence of a progressive development of two divergent but ultimately compatible tendencies which, it appears safe to say, will continue to characterize the evolution of pediatrics. The first refers to the need for separateness of pediatric training and facilities. The second is the rising needs of the adolescent and of the family unit, and the necessity for long-term study of health and disease which must bring the children's unit closer to the adult unit.

It is of interest that in these contrasting tendencies surgery has necessarily presented an increasingly vital need for in-patient facilities while the medical aspects of pediatrics are tending more and more toward out-patient facilities, preventive factors, long-term care and home care.

When one also reviews the teaching pediatric units throughout the world it is impressive that the formula for their origin and growth has generally followed the attitude toward pediatric centers of the era in which they were built. Additions or rearrangement of buildings or major moves have depended more on personalities and the provincial ideas of local authorities than on adequate studies of pediatric trends.

But if I see the future trends of pediatrics correctly the explosion of knowledge which is part of, and bears directly on, this specialty must bring the biologic sequence of pediatric instruction in medical education into the commanding position it inevitably must occupy. The examples of this sequence are crowding to the forefront of medical investigation. One illustrative case is the topsy-turvy position in which psychiatry often finds itself. One of the most cogent proofs to my knowledge of the subconscious lies in the findings Wilder Penfield has presented of the results of probing with a fine-needle electrode the temporal area related to memory while the patient is fully conscious—a process by which the adult patient recalls whole areas and scenes of childhood, even bits of conversation and forgotten languages, which are apparently beyond recall without such probing. These results, as well as others, fully corroborate the possibility of recall by association of infant, childhood or adolescent experiences which are profoundly important to adult behavior. In the normal biologic sequence the child psychiatrist and the pediatrician interested in psychologic pediatrics have been asking why we should not start with infancy and childhood and if possible watch the development of those physical or psychological events or disturbances that compose the subconscious of later years. Perhaps even psychoses as well as neuroses might be avoided or at least better understood when they are incipient. Also how exciting it will be for the pediatrician to explore a preventive area which already in many situations has opened far more hopeful prospects than the treatment of the seriously disturbed adult. The exploration of such problems in children, which inevitably involve the entire family, may in itself preserve the parents as well from crippling neuroses secondary to their child's problem. Should not psychiatric teaching, then, start with its natural biologic beginning, the brain of the infant, the child and the adolescent, and proceed from the simpler to the more complex, from the few reactions to the many?

To ask this question is to suggest the wealth of pediatric opportunity.

Another opportunity in such biologic sequence is the joining of the basic sciences with pediatrics in the exploding field of genetics—an area in which pediatrics has an unexcelled opportunity and in which the basic sciences and pediatrics should jointly construct the bridge from the former into the early beginnings of clinical medicine. Again, the opportunities for studying the possible salvage of individuals from handicaps and crippling disabilities could well excite the imagination of anyone considering pediatrics as a lifework.

Medicine in the future will depend to a major extent on pediatrics for the elucidation of endocrine problems in their earliest and simplest phases—for the understanding of the nutritional and genetic backgrounds of early atherosclerosis, of kidney disease, of rheumatic fever and crippling heart disease, in their simplest form.

No specialty has as great an opportunity to study basic immunologic mechanisms and allergies in the virgin soil of infancy and childhood and in the production of antibodies and immunization with antigens—the homotransplant in infancy and the entire area of immunologic tolerance upon which so much of the future studies in immunology depends. Malignant disease well illustrates the manner in which gross pathology and surgery are yielding quite properly to biochemistry, microscopic pathology and microbiology, and here the high pediatric incidence of neoplasms (the second highest cause of death between 4 and 12 years) has caused effort to be concentrated in this area. Chemotherapy with scarce materials is highly suitable for children. Such diseases as acute leukemia have their highest incidence at this age; thus malignancy can be studied in its most uncomplicated form, as it occurs in infants and children.

I have noted above in order:

The maturing and mellowing influence on perceptive persons of work in the field of children and youth, in medical care, as well as for others skilled in this area.

The high social value—the altruistic and philanthropic aspects of love of mankind—existing to a larger degree among most of those entering pediatrics in medical schools as compared with most other medical students who appear to be deficient in this value. The reasons for the historically delayed interest in and development of pediatrics and its accelerating significance, both in the basic biologic sciences and in all of medicine, which is the result of a gradual acknowledgment of its position in the natural biologic sequence from the embryo to the adult.

The unity of the developing studies of the preclinical sciences on cellular processes—unicellular as compared with multicellular—being succeeded by a growing unity of the clinical departments in educational emphasis—again with an increasing emphasis on the natural biologic sequence, starting with the young.

How do these 4 brief summations and their elaboration above bear on academic pediatrics and pediatric practice? In the short space of a single presentation one can best concentrate on the philosophical and historical perspective and point but briefly to the present and the future of pediatrics.

ACADEMIC PEDIATRICS

"Yet all experience is an arch wherethro' gleams that untravell'd world whose margin fades forever and forever when I move." In the field of academic work one may consider the supporting pillars of the arch as teaching and patient care, joined together by the keystone of the arch, research. The more perfect the construction of the arch, the clearer the vision and the better the frame of reference for exploring the unknown.

Clinical investigation began when pediatrics was slowly separating from the rest of medicine at the end of the 19th century. Abraham Jacobi, a revolutionary follower of Carl Schurz, bridged the gap between the already advancing pediatrics on the continent—chiefly in Germany—and American medicine. The prime founder of the American Pediatric Society in 1888, he also became president of the American Medical Association, and the medical culture he brought from the continent stimulated an increasing interest in the study of infants and children. Emmett Holt, Sr., and a number of other able clinicians, rapidly developed the entire field of clinical pediatrics in academic centers, but it was not until the first full-time chair of pediatrics was created at Johns Hopkins University under John Howland in 1913 that the golden age of pediatrics began in the United States. The joining of laboratory and clinical investigation was the key to this development, and its leavening influence was spread through the other academic centers by a corps of such able investigators and teachers as Park, Gamble, Powers, Blackfan, Marriott, Kramer, Davison and others.

The vital importance of research to pediatric practice as well as academic pediatrics is perhaps best illustrated by the content of presentations before all of the pediatric societies. Not only in the American Pediatric Society and its younger counterpart, the Society for Pediatric Research, but in the American Academy of Pediatrics it is rare that a paper is presented that does not outline or summarize one of the manifold

aspects of academic research in this field. Those who carry
their knowledge, remedies and vaccines from door to door or
utilize them in their offices often forget or overlook the thousands of men and women in clinical and laboratory research
upon whose accomplishments the practitioners are depending
and from whose efforts their incomes are essentially derived—
incomes considerably larger than those of a legion of investigators, past and present, who have made possible the effective
work of those in practice.

The growing emphasis and effort placed in schools of medicine on the young growing organism and its problems in
pediatrics, preventive medicine, public health and general
practice with respect to clinical investigation, teaching and
laboratory research offer the student, the intern and the
resident a fertile field for his academic interests. It is also of
interest that training in pediatrics frequently has been a step-
ping stone to the field of preventive medicine and public
health, to school health work, and to administrative positions
in schools of medicine.

Perhaps the outstanding fact in the actual conduct of pediatrics, both in the academic field and in practice, is the developing trend of all clinical specialties toward group practice. All academic centers are essentially examples of group
practice in their care of patients. It is to be hoped that in the
future the examples of the few academic pioneers who have
unified their fiscal arrangements, just as the large private
group practices do, to prevent marked inequality of income,
and thereby of power and control, will extend throughout the
country to all academic centers. The length of time that pediatricians must spend with families to satisfy the required con-
siderate handling of both the young and their parents and the
obvious difficulty young parents have in adequately paying
for such pediatric services warrants mature consideration by
the medical profession as a whole. The social value and sense
of social responsibility of the pediatrician have been regarded
as satisfying his lack of income. However, the inequality of
income has been too great. Those pediatricians who at present

receive the largest incomes do so only by neglecting the basic premises upon which modern pediatrics must be practiced—the complete medical care of the growing organism, physically, psychologically and ethically in close association with the family unit. These men with largest incomes too often skip superficially from case to case while the mature enjoyment of the complete practice of pediatrics escapes them.

In the training of students, interns and residents the aim of pediatric teaching has been increasingly to prepare the pediatrician by group practice in the academic center for group practice in the community, whether in small pediatric groups that work closely with urban or suburban hospitals where the other specialists or general practitioners are available, or in larger group practices where all of the branches of medicine converge into a single unit, pooling income and facilities, and often extending their advantages to prepayment plans for families attached to their groups. Prepayment for physicians' services strongly supports the interest of both physicians and families in prevention and in the promotion of health, as increasingly demonstrated by such groups as the Health Insurance Plan of New York City.

A study by the U. S. Public Health Service showed that from 1946 to 1959 the number of group medical practice units in the United States more than tripled while about 16,500 physicians, or 10 per cent of all those in active practice, were members of such groups in 1959.

To carry out this type or any type of pediatric practice it is essential that the student take 3 years of pediatric training after graduation and 2 additional years in practice in order to qualify for the examinations and certification by the American Board of Pediatrics.

The "new" pediatrics or the "comprehensive" pediatrics which has been discussed in recent pediatric publications merely indicates the maturing of pediatric practice with the realization by pediatricians that the care of the infant, the child and the adolescent must be related to the entire family milieu; that, for example, juvenile delinquency is directly related to the earliest years when adequate positive handling by the physician, among others, could well have prevented the twig from bending in the wrong direction. If bent at the wrong time in development it may perpetuate a wayward growth or even break, or it may spring back. The pediatrician almost invariably is consulted about early deviations in the behavior of children before the minister, the priest, or the rabbi. His responsibility and opportunity in this area are as yet but dimly discerned. As Sir James Spence has expressed it, a new Vesalius or Sydenham is needed to point up by careful research in this area when and what are the skills to be required.

In the final analysis the basic qualifications for a pediatrician are direct and simple: he must be a physician who has deep affection for and interest in the young and a feeling for his stewardship in supporting not only these youthful apprentices to life but their parents as well.

REFERENCES

1. Speech of Charles Dickens, Esq. as Chairman at the Dinner on behalf of the Hospital for Sick Children at Freemason's Hall, Feb. 9, 1858.

2. Differential Characteristics of Student Bodies—Implications for the Study of Medical Education—Helen Hofer Gee, Director of Research Association of American Medical Colleges.

CLARENCE S. LIVINGOOD, M.D.

*Director, Department of Dermatology at the
Henry Ford Hospital*

5

Dermatology

The reasons for choosing a given specialty as a career in medicine are fairly complex. In this discussion on dermatology, no attempt will be made to undertake an intensive analysis of all of the positive factors that would influence a young physician to be a dermatologist, because to do so would present the prejudiced point of view of one who is already in this field of medicine, and who, so to speak, must validate his own choice.

One acceptable approach in describing what it means to be a dermatologist is to review in some detail the history and development of the specialty with the thought that, in this manner, the reader will be oriented in regard to the scope of dermatology in the over-all practice of medicine, the training required for specialization in this field, the contributions that dermatologists have made to medical progress, the opportunities for investigative work in the field, the service that it offers to the individual and society, and the rewards and satisfactions that it holds for those engaged in it.

We know from the earliest medical writings that cutaneous diseases have always constituted one of the major interests of medicine. In the Ebers Papyrus, which was written 3500 years ago, and in the "Hippocratic Collection," a group of volumes printed about 100 years after the death of Hippocrates, there are numerous references to diseases involving the skin. The early Arabian physicians, especially Avicenna (A.D. 980-1037), described many diseases of the skin including warts, pigmentation disorders, scar formation, carbuncles, ichthyosis, impetigo, anthrax and pediculi. This is understandable since the skin is the organ of the body most available for study, but also this attention to skin diseases in the early writings reflects a relatively high incidence.

The dividing of medicine into various specialties was gradual, starting during the early part of the nineteenth century, and accelerating during the latter part of the century. Dermatology is one of the specialties that had its origin as a separate and distinct branch of medicine during this period. Primarily, the pioneers in the specialty were concerned with outlining a satisfactory classification of skin diseases; it is appropriate to refer to this early period of dermatology as "the classification and morphologic era."

The first modern text on dermatology was written in 1777 by a Frenchman, Antoine Charles Lorry (1723-83) and essentially this treatise dealt with classification. Also Lorry was the first to recognize the systemic manifestations of drug eruptions. Thirty-one years later, an Englishman, Robert Willan (1757-1812) wrote a more comprehensive book which was illustrated in color and which summarized his efforts in classifying and defining skin diseases. In 1845, Ferdinand von Hebra (1816-80) of Vienna published his work on cutaneous diseases which was based on pathologic and anatomic features of dermatoses. Hebra was a brilliant teacher, a tireless worker, a great clinician, and a forceful personality. He was the greatest dermatologist of the century and probably it is appropriate to consider him the founder of modern dermatology.

There are a great many other men who contributed to the development of the specialty in its early days. In France, Jean Louis Marc Alibert (1767-1837) founded the first center for the study of skin diseases, the Hôpital St. Louis; he too, in 1829, wrote a treatise on skin diseases, in which he summarized his own ideas on classification, and included original descriptions of mycosis fungoides and keloid. Two other eminent pioneer French dermatologists were Jean Darier (1856-1938), who achieved great international stature as the author of an eight-volume work on skin diseases, and Raymond Sabouraud (1864-1938) who made extensive studies of mycotic skin infections and was the founder of modern mycology. In Germany, Paul Gerson Unna (1850-1929) applied fixed-tissue pathologic interpretation in advancing the depth and breadth of dermatology. He published important works on the histopathology of the skin and on the treatment of skin diseases. Unna's gelatin boot is still the best single modality for the treatment of stasis ulcers.

The first book on dermatology published in the United States was, "A Synopsis of Diseases of the Skin," by Noah Worcester (1812-1847) of Harvard. James White (1833-1916) of Boston, Louis A. Duhring (1845-1913) of Philadelphia and George Henry Fox (1846-1937) of New York, are only three of numerous eminent pioneer American dermatologists, whose original contributions, teaching and writing had a profound influence on the early growth and stature of the specialty in the United States.

When dermatology first became established as a specialty of medicine it included syphilis, and until a few years ago the appropriate name for the specialty was Dermatology and Syphilology. Thus, for example, until a short time ago, the **AMA Archives of Dermatology** was the **Archives of Dermatology and Syphilology.** In addition, with the exception of gonorrhea, the other venereal diseases, lymphogranuloma venereum, chancroid, and granuloma inguinale are in the dermatologist's domain.

The three leading contributions to the study of syphilis during the early part of the present century were made in the laboratory by Schaudinn (1871-1906) of Germany, who discovered the *Spirochaeta pallida;* by Wassermann (1866-1925) of Germany, who discovered the blood test for syphilis, the well-known "Wassermann reaction"; and by Paul Ehrlich (1845-1915) who in 1909 discovered a specific antisyphilitic therapeutic agent which he called salvarsan. Most of the studies relating to the clinical manifestations of syphilis, the course of the disease and its modern treatment have been made by dermatologists. John H. Stokes (1885-_____) Emeritus Professor of Dermatology and Syphilology of the University of Pennsylvania, deserves special recognition as one of the outstanding clinical syphilologists of the past half century. His book on syphilis (the last edition with the collaboration of Beerman and Ingraham) is one of the all-time classics of medical literature. One of the dramatic therapeutic advances of the last two decades was the introduction of penicillin for the treatment of syphilis. As a direct result there has been a marked decrease in prevalence, and the treatment of the disease has been simplified. As recently as ten to twenty years ago, most of the teaching clinics were truly departments of dermatology and syphilology and a significant percentage of the patients who were seen in these clinics had syphilis or other venereal diseases. Syphilis is still an integral part of the dermatologist's training but at the present time the management of syphilis and other venereal diseases represents only a minor part of his practice.

The evolutionary development of dermatology from the morphologic and classification era to the present functional era has been accompanied by the emergence of the specialty as a clinical science. A sketchy review of the high points of this development which follows makes it apparent that no other specialty except, perhaps, internal medicine, calls for as much knowledge in other clinical fields and in the basic sciences.

As noted previously, the first step in this development was the invention of a nomenclature and the application of the objective descriptive discipline to skin lesions. The training and experience of the dermatologist results in the development of remarkably accurate observation and deduction to the point that often the expert assessment of the morphologic characteristics and the distribution of the lesions makes it possible to arrive at a definitive diagnosis on initial examination of the patient.

The next step was the application of fixed-tissue pathologic interpretation. Hebra, and later Unna, established the foundations of dermatopathology. The availability of the skin for biopsy, and repeated biopsy if necessary, facilitates, confirms or tends to rule out diagnoses, frequently in a very definite manner, so that in this regard the practice of dermatology is on a more scientific basis than perhaps any other specialty. Dermatopathology has always been an important part of the training program of a dermatologist, and for the most part the development of this specialized field of pathology has been within the province of the dermatologist, not the pathologist.

Early in the developmental period of the specialty, Sabouraud made his monumental contributions* in descriptive mycology. In 1912, J. Jadassohn first elaborated the dermatophytid concept and some years later in a series of brilliant investigations, Bloch and his colleagues identified and demonstrated the relation of trichophytin to the problems of allergization.

It is important to emphasize that in addition to their work on morphology and classification, some of these early eminent men did basic investigative work which not only had a profound effect in advancing our fund of knowledge in regard to skin diseases but also influenced significantly the progress of medicine in general. Four of the great men in this category were Paul Unna, J. Jadassohn, Jean Darier and later Bruno Bloch, who were dermatologists with a broad background of knowledge in the basic sciences, tireless workers in the laboratory and equally important, they stimulated and guided their numerous pupils and junior associates in the application of laboratory methods in dermatologic research.

Gardner Hopkins, Fred Weidman, George Lewis, and J. Walter Wilson are only four of numerous American dermatologists whose names are associated with clinical and laboratory investigative work in the field of medical mycology

---

• "Les trichophytes humaines" (1894) and "Les teignes" (1910).

both in respect to the superficial and the deep mycoses, which have cutaneous manifestations. The dermatologist is unique in that he is the only clinical specialist who is required to have intensive laboratory work in mycology during his residency training period.

Much of the pioneer work in the use of roentgenology and radium for the treatment of malignant tumors of the skin, lymphomatous disease, and various dermatoses has been done by dermatologists. Pusey, Miescher, and Keinboch were three of these pioneers. These fundamental contributions include the development of dosage schedules, epilation technics for the treatment of tinea capitis, the concept of the erythema dose, absorption studies, and exit dose factors. MacKee and Cipollaro deserve special recognition for their excellent book on this subject.

A review of the achievements of dermatologists in developing an understanding of the allergic mechanisms of cutaneous diseases makes it evident that the specialty has an important stake in the fields of allergy and immunology. The patch test, so useful for the detection of allergic contact dermatitis, was described by J. Jadassohn as early as 1894 and in later years was further developed by Bruno Bloch and his co-workers in Europe and Marion Sulzberger and his associates in the United States. Darier, J. Jadassohn, Bloch, Sulzberger, W. Jadassohn, Haxthausen, Frei, R. L. Mayer, Baer, Rostenberg, Urbach, Peck and Kligman are only some of the dermatologists associated with investigative work on the problems of distant allergic responses (tuberculid, dermatophytid and other "id" eruptions) emanating from localized infection, epidermal sensitization, localized sensitivity, cross sensitization, eczematous sensitization, atopy, drug allergy and tissue, serums and cell antibodies. Almost all of the extensive investigative work in the field of occupational dermatoses has been done by dermatologists. Prosser-White, L. Schwartz, J. Downing, Klauder, Peck and Birmingham are some of the contributors to our fund of knowledge concerning this important segment of occupational diseases.

Dermatologists have been responsible for some of the most significant diagnostic and therapeutic developments in a long list of systemic diseases with cutaneous manifestations, especially lupus erythematosus, sarcoidosis, scleroderma, dermatomyositis, lipid diseases, pigmentary disorders, porphyria, cutaneous tuberculosis, leprosy and syphilis. The names associated with these contributions are so numerous that it is impossible to list all of them. Because of limitations of space, comments will be restricted to only a few of these diseases. Almost a century ago, Kaposi first recognized the systemic manifestations of lupus erythematosus and a short time later J. Jadassohn reported on the frequency of kidney involvement, fever, and mucous membrane involvement in systemic lupus erythematosus. O'Leary, Michelson, Brunsting, Curtis and Haserick are only five of many dermatologists who have written extensively on lupus erythematosus, dermatomyositis and scleroderma. Haserick isolated the LE cell factor, responsible for the LE phenomenon; he and Hargraves described the LE test simultaneously. Most of the work on light sensitivity has been done by dermatologists—Lamb and his coworkers, Kesten and others. Many years ago both the cutaneous and the systemic manifestations of sarcoidosis as well as its immunologic reactions, were described by Boeck, Darier, Besnier, Roussy, Schaumann, Lewandowsky and Jadassohn and more recently, the Kveim test for sarcoidosis was developed in the dermatology clinic of Danbolt in Norway. Grutz, Urbach, Oppenheim, Curtis and his coworkers, and Lever are some of the numerous dermatologists who were responsible for advances in our knowledge of lipid diseases.

A very important and significant development in dermatology since World War II is that an increasing number of investigators with broad basic training and interests, most of them accomplished dermatologists, are devoting themselves with imagination and success to the application of the electron microscope, capillary microscopy, histochemistry, tissue culture, and other technics, to the investigation of derma-

tologic problems.* Static anatomy and pathology have been
amplified by functional anatomy and pathology. Representative examples of these studies include Winkleman's
work on the sensory nerve endings of the skin; the histo-
chemical studies of Mescon, Steigleder and others; the work
of Hermann Pinkus in the study of mitoses by stripping of
the skin; Tzanck's cytodiagnostic studies; the use of the
electron microscope by Blank and his co-workers in describing histologic details of the epidermis; and Funan Hu's application of tissue culture technics in the study of the melanocyte
and other cells of the epidermis. Also advances have been
made in our understanding of bacteriology of the normal
and abnormal skin, especially by Pillsbury and his associates,
and in virology by Blank and his co-workers and by Wheeler
and Cawley.

An important factor in the accelerated rate of the development of the functional era in dermatology during the past
fifteen years has been the unparalleled surge of interest in
cutaneous physiology and biochemistry of the skin.

The list of dermatologists who are using these basic disciplines in the study of normal and abnormal function of
the skin is such a long one that it is impossible to cite all of
their names. Particular recognition is due Stephen Rothman
of Chicago not only because of the important contributions
that he and his group have made in many areas of these
fields of investigation but also because of his classic book,
"Physiology and Biochemistry of the Skin," which has become
one of the standard textbooks for the student of dermatology.

With apologies to those whose work is not included, com-

---

* Numerous factors have contributed to the postwar emphasis on basic research in dermatology departments throughout the country. Two of these deserve special comment: (1) The excellent annual meetings of the Society of
Investigative Dermatology, which have served as a forum for the presentation
and discussion of these studies and (2) the very important and indeed dominant role of Dr. Donald M. Pillsbury in obtaining the support of scientists in
other fields of medicine for increased facilities for basic research in dermatology; the direct result of his efforts in this regard has been increasing government financial support of such research.

pilation of a partial list of the advances in this area which have been made in this country since World War II, includes Shelley and Arthur's concept of the enzymatic basis for itching, the evaluation of the problem of sweat retention by Shelley, Sulzberger and Hermann, the physiology of the eccrine sweat glands by Lobitz and Dobson, Shelley, and Hermann, the physiology of the apocrine sweat glands by Shelley and Perry, studies of the pH of the skin by Blank, the work of Lever, Curtis, Rukivina and Bloch on lipid diseases, the isolation of melanocyte stimulating hormone by Lerner and his associates, elucidation of the pigment metabolism by Fitzpatrick and Lerner, the contributions to our knowledge of the biochemistry of the epidermis by Flesch and Esoda, the isolation of the protein, cryoglobulin, by Lerner, and the investigation of the role of properiden in host resistance to fungus infections and other diseases by Sternberg, McNall and Newcomer.

This interest in basic research has not resulted in the neglect of morphologic observation and clinical study. Indeed, because of the accessibility of the skin, one of the characteristics of research in dermatology has been the successful correlation of function and structure, perhaps more so than in any other specialty.

This brief review of some of the pertinent historical facts regarding the development of dermatology from its early beginnings to its present scientific dynamic status makes it evident that the dermatologist does not confine his attention to the skin itself. As stated in the beginning of this chapter, he must have a broad medical base, for no other specialty, except perhaps internal medicine, calls for so much knowledge in other fields. Callaway* in his excellent article on "Contributions by Dermatology to the Progress of Medicine" has outlined the development and evaluation of dermatology through the years, and in a very lucid and accurate manner summaries the present status of the specialty as follows:

---

* Callaway, J. Lamar: A.M.A. Archives of Dermatology *80*:649-662, 1959.

"Dermatology today might more concisely be described as cutaneous medicine. Although the morphologic characteristics of cutaneous lesions, readily visible to the naked eye (or studied with magnification), often offer a practical solution to the problem, the dermatologist's concept is never limited to the integument and often involves the evaluation of bone marrow, lymph nodes, endocrine glands, various immunologic studies, biochemical analyses, as well as scrapings, cultures (mycologic and bacterial), and biopsies of the skin. Curtis, Sutton Jr., O'Leary, Stokes and many others have for years stressed the importance of the whole individual and not the skin alone. Today, the dermatologist needs and, indeed, has a background as profound as the internist."

The tremendous scope of dermatology becomes apparent when one considers the complexity and multiple functions of the skin and its appendages; its potentialities for injury; its frequent, almost daily, contact with potential irritants and allergens; the numerous benign and malignant new growths that may originate in it and its appendages; the vast number of diseases that involve the skin primarily; the importance of pruritus as a symptom; the cosmetic implications of skin lesions; the tendency for a high percentage of drug reactions to involve the skin; and the fact that almost all systemic disorders may have cutaneous signs and symptoms. Add to these considerations the fact that dermatology is to some degree a surgical specialty as well as a medical specialty, in that minor surgery of the skin is in the domain of the dermatologist, and it becomes even more obvious that the physician who selects dermatology as his specialty will find that he has elected to follow a challenging career with many different facets.

The great diversity and the importance of the diseases involving the skin and mucous membranes, which primarily are the concern of the dermatologist, are not realized by the vast majority of the medical profession. This is in part due to the fact that in most of the medical schools of this country, the curricula neglect the teaching of the theory and practice of dermatology. Because of this, there are numerous misconceptions regarding dermatology, which, as Sulzberger and Baer* have stated, "are based on false notions concerning such important matters as the nomenclature of dermatology, the number and the nature of the diseases it deals with, its diagnostic and therapeutic problems, its practical methods and results and its past substantial contributions and uncalculable potentialities for basic medical teaching and fundamental research."

The fact is that diseases of the skin and its related mucous membranes represent an estimated 8 to 12 per cent of the practice of medicine. There are nineteen departments of dermatology in the medical centers of the United States, which average more than 1000 out-patient visits a month, and in six institutions the total number is more than 20,000 each year. The physician who chooses dermatology as his specialty can be assured that he will not have a paucity of patients, even if he elects to practice in a community with a population as small as 25,000 to 30,000 individuals.

Experience accumulated during World War II brought into focus the importance of dermatologic diseases as a cause of partial and total disability. In some military hospitals, skin diseases accounted for 20 per cent or more of the total admissions and a similar proportion on out patient "sick-call" had dermatologic complaints. With the exception of neuropsychiatric disturbances, more American soldiers were evacuated to the United States from tropical overseas theaters because of skin diseases than for any other group of disorders, and throughout the war they exceeded the number of evacuees because of battle injuries. At the beginning of the war, dermatology as a specialty was practically non-existent in the Armed Forces. By the end of the war, dermatology had become established as one of the major specialties in military

---

* Sulzberger, Marion B., and Baer, Rudolph L.: Some Common Misconceptions Regarding Dermatology; Year Book of Dermatology and Syphilology (Chicago), The Year Book Publishers, Inc., 1947, p. 5-32. (This excellent article should be required reading for all medical educators.)

hospitals and since then this emphasis has continued, and excellent dermatology training centers have been established in a number of Armed Forces teaching hospitals.

It is evident to the reader at this stage of our discussion that dermatology is not an easy specialty in which a physician can qualify by taking a brief post-graduate course. In this country, the American Board of Dermatology and Syphilology, founded in 1932, was one of the earliest of the boards formed for the purpose of defining qualifications for specializing in the various fields of medicine and certifying those who meet those standards. To qualify, the physician must have three years of formal training in an approved institution, and this training must include the fundamentals of dermatopathology, mycology, biochemistry and physiology of the skin, immunology, allergy, and physics of radiation therapy. During his training he will gradually acquire the power of accurate observation and deduction to a degree that usually is not approached in any other field of medicine. He will learn the importance of the whole individual and not the skin alone and he will acquire the broad general medical background essential in evaluating the many patients whose cutaneous lesions are manifestations of systemic disease. He will learn to correlate laboratory and clinical findings, to estimate prognosis in a surprisingly accurate manner and to correlate function and structure. He will learn the principles of therapy and in the process he will learn that, unfortunately, some dermatologic patients do die, that they may awaken you in the middle of the night and that a very high proportion do get well, providing they are treated in an expert manner —indeed, the response to proper treatment is most gratifying in a high percentage of cases and there is no more grateful group of patients. Also, the embryo dermatologist in training will find that these three years will be the most stimulating and rewarding years of his professional life.

In conclusion, if one seeks an increasing challenge, unlimited opportunities for basic and clinical research, wide diversity in practice, a continuing opportunity to test one's own discernment and skill, the fellowship of lifelong enthusiasts who are never bored, and the gratitude of multitudinous sufferers, one will find his rightful place in dermatology. If one is looking for an easy specialty, and a sure and undemanding financial return, he should not choose dermatology nor indeed any other branch of medicine.

H. HOUSTON MERRITT, M.D.

Professor of Neurology at Columbia University

6

Neurology

Neurology emerged as a special branch of internal medicine approximately a century ago. The nervous system was the subject of study by ancient physicians, but the concept of humors and vital spirits prevailed in the writings of Hippocrates and Galen. Convulsive seizures and headache were the two neurological symptoms that received most attention in the writings of ancient physicians. With the Renaissance, neurology began to advance on the foundation of a scientific anatomy in the 16th century by Leonardo da Vinci and Vesalius. Further advances were made in the 17th century by Willis, Vieussens, van Leeuwenhock, Pacchioni and others. These men paved the way for the studies in the 18th century that culminated in such fine atlases of the nervous system as that of Soemmerring.

The development of the concepts of the physiology of the central nervous system paralleled to a great extent the growth of knowledge of anatomy. Signal advances were not made, however, until the 19th century. The studies of such men as Sir Charles Bell, Johannes Muller, E. H. Weber, A. V. Waller, Du Bois-Reymond, Gustav Fritsch, Eduard Hitzig, J. C. Dalton, David Ferrier, John Hughlings Jackson, and others, culminated in the modern neurophysiology typified by the writings of Sir Charles S. Sherrington.

On the background of these advances in anatomy and physiology, neurology began to emerge as a clinical specialty in the middle and the latter parts of the 19th century. Guillaume B. A. Duchenne is generally credited with being the founder of modern clinical neurology. He was followed in France by J. M. Charcot, Pierre Marie, Josef F. F. Babinski and J. J. Dejerine; in Germany, by M. H. Romberg, W. H. Erb, C. F. O. Wesphal and H. Oppenheim; in England, by John Hughlings Jackson, D. Ferrier, William R. Gowers, H. C. Bastian, Henry Head and S. A. Kinnier Wilson.

Although the pathology of the central nervous system was studied in the 17th and the 18th centuries, neuropathology did not come of age until the first part of the present century. The names of a few who have contributed to the development of neuropathology include Alois Alzheimer, Max Bielschowsky, Constantin von Economo, Alfons Jacob, Franz Nissl, Walter Spielmeyer and Karl Weigert, of Germany; Raymon Y. Cajal and Pio del Rio Hortega, of Spain; Ettore Marchiafava and Giovanni Mingazzini, of Italy; Jean Cruveilhier, of France; Georges Marinesco, of Rumania; J. Godwin Greenfield, of England; and J. H. Globus and W. B. Hassin, of the United States.

Neurology in the United States was born in the period of the Civil War. In 1862 W. A. Hammond, Surgeon General of the Union Forces, established in Philadelphia a special military hospital for nervous diseases. This was just two years after the founding of the National Hospital for Paralyzed and Epileptics, at Queen Square, in London. An independent chair in neurology was established in 1871 at the College of Physicians and Surgeons of Columbia University in New York, with Edouard Seguin as Professor of Diseases of the Nervous System. In Philadelphia, at the University of Pennsylvania, H. C. Wood was appointed professor of diseases of the nervous system in 1876. In Boston, James J. Putnam was made lecturer, in 1872, but neurology was not separated from medicine at Harvard until 1895.

On the firm background of anatomy, physiology and pathology, neurology has advanced in the United States from its modest beginnings in three medical schools. At the present time there are independent departments or specialized sub-departments of neurology in most of the schools of this country. The American Neurological Association has grown from a membership of 35 in 1875, to over 400 in 1960; and the recently founded American Academy of Neurology has a membership of more than 2000. In addition, there are special societies for neuropathology, neurophysiology, electro-encephalography and neurochemistry. More than a dozen journals dealing with clinical neurology or with various aspects of neurology are published in the English language. A World Federation of Neurology has recently been founded with approximately 8000 members from all countries of the world.

In its early years, neurology was linked with internal medicine. With the development of the new specialty of psychiatry, it was only natural that neurologists, as students of the nervous system, were in the forefront of this new field. A new type of specialist, the neuropsychiatrist, was born. With the rapid growth of psychiatry during the first three decades of this century, neurology slipped into the background. Specialists in neuropsychiatry were trained in both psychiatry and neurology, but the emphasis in their training was in psychiatry. It gradually became evident that it was not possible, with but few exceptions, for a physician to be proficient in both neurology and psychiatry. The scant training in neurology made the neuropsychiatrist of little help to his medical colleague in the management of a patient with organic diseases of the nervous system, and the magnitude of the number of patients with minor and major psychiatric disturbances absorbed most of the efforts of the neuropsychiatrists. This, together with the growth of knowledge in both fields, made it obvious that separation of the two specialties was necessary. In the first few years following the formation of the American Board of Psychiatry and Neurology, more than half of the candidates were certified in both specialties. At the present time, double certification is sought by less than 1 per cent of the candidates, although some training in both fields is required of all candidates. It should be noted, however, that the specialty of neuropsychiatry continues to flourish in many of the countries on the European continent.

A number of factors are responsible for the rebirth of neurology in this country. Among these are the growth of specialties in general; the relative increase in the importance of chronic diseases; the formation of lay health organizations dedicated to the improvement of the care of patients with specific diseases through the establishment of adequate clinical and research facilities; and the creation of the National Institute of Neurological Diseases and Blindness in the National Institutes of Health in the United States Public Health Service. All of these factors increased the number of patients who sought the attention of the practicing neurologist and made opportunities available for a career in research or teaching.

It is difficult to determine what factors attract a medical student to select a field of specialization. The temperament of the student, the personality of his instructors, opportunities that present themselves and many other unknown factors play a role. Early in his career, the student is exposed to the intricacies of the anatomy and the physiology of the nervous system. The use of polysyllabic terms in the basic sciences and in the clinic may have a tendency to divert some students from the fields. Fortunately, teachers of the present day have found that neurology can be taught without unduly complex terminology, and that the examination of the nervous system need not be a time-consuming laborious procedure. On the other hand, the preciseness with which abnormalities of function of the nervous system can be determined and the diagnosis of disease established is appealing to the analytical mind.

One of the factors that had for many years unfavorably influenced the student in the selection of neurology was the oft-repeated statement that it was a specialty that was "long on diagnosis but short on therapy." This criticism is voiced less often at present. The opportunities for therapy of patients with neurological disease are about equal to those of any other specialty. With the conquest of the infectious diseases, medicine in general is confronted with an increasing number of patients with long-term illnesses in whom the course of treatment is prolonged.

The opportunities for the practitioner of neurology of today are great. He is responsible for the care of a vast number of patients with a great variety of diseases, including the acute and the chronic infections of the nervous system, cerebral vascular diseases, epilepsy, migraine, multiple sclerosis, brain and spinal cord tumors, myasthenia gravis, muscular dystrophy, various so-called heredodegenerative diseases, congenital or inborn structural or metabolic diseases. Diagnostic aids available to him make it possible to determine accurately the nature of the organic or functional lesion in the nervous system. For many of his patients he has a specific curative therapy. For others, he has methods of treatment that alleviate or control the process to a degree sufficient to restore the individual to his status as a productive citizen. He can call on his neurosurgical colleagues in the treatment of patients with operable tumors of the nervous system amenable to surgery, and on the radiotherapist for the treatment of other types of tumors. The physiotherapist, too, is of invaluable aid in the rehabilitation of patients with static lesions.

For the academic neurologist, the opportunities are greater today than at any time in the history of the specialist. The number of teachers in medical schools has increased greatly during the past few years, and the opportunities for research in the basic sciences and clinical fields are unlimited. The challenge to conquer any one of a number of neurological diseases is a great stimulus, and new methods of investigation are of sufficient promise to attract the promising student to a career in neurology.

JOHN ROMANO, M.D.
Professor of Psychiatry at the University of Rochester

7

Psychiatry

Introduction.   Psychiatry is the most personal of the medical disciplines. For this and other reasons I believe it to be the most interesting. Whereas it is a medical specialty in that many psychiatrists devote and restrict themselves to the diagnosis and treatment of the mentally sick, it is more than this. More than during any previous period in medical history, serious and persistent attempts are being made to accumulate the primary data that one day may be established as a basic science of human biology. Toward this objective of the scientific humanization of biology, psychiatry is taking its part. Together with the social sciences, it has begun to make systematic inquiries into many areas of human behavior, both individual and group, previously either totally disregarded by medical science or, if considered, done so more or less exclusively with empirical means and in artistic and intuitive terms.

Not only man's body, but his mind, his emotions and their reciprocal effects on his body have become the legitimate concern of scientific medicine. Modern psychiatry is interested in man's relations with his family and other groups; in the continuum between health and disease; in the nature of the bonds between patient and physician; in the psychology and sociology of the sick person, whether he be acutely ill, convalescent, disabled or deformed; in the social set of hospitals and other institutions; and in the relations between those who share in the study, care and treatment of the sick.

Modern psychiatry is also interested in learning more about those genic and experiential factors, inextricably interwoven, which lead in time to the emergence of man's increasing capacity for adult, interdependent, responsible behavior from his incredibly parasitic infantile beginnings. It is concerned in learning more about the ubiquitous normative emotional crises that occur among the members of each human family; crises which, if unresolved or managed unwisely, may lead to disease and disability in one or more members of the family. The basic concepts of health and disease properly command the attention of modern medical scientists. In this, modern psychiatry may contribute its share, particularly in conjunction with its colleagues who are currently investigating the biochemical, neurophysiologic, behavioral and social aspects of the dynamic steady state of the individual organism within its environment.

Modern psychiatry is attempting to define more precisely what it is that constitutes mental illness. What are the zones of healthy behavior? To which degree are these judgments universal, to which are they dependent upon values set by a society at a certain time in its history. It has become increasingly concerned with ideas of prevention and this has led inevitably and most properly to the need for more precise epidemiologic data, to incidence and prevalence studies of illness and social disability in large and small human populations. Treatment of the sick is its oldest heritage and is responsible for its name, psychiatry. How effective are our therapeutic interventions? How successful are our currently used psychologic, social, pharmacologic and physical measures with their various combinations in relieving the distress of our patients?

These are the matters that interest and engage psychiatry. They pose the questions that must be answered if psychiatry is to make a major contribution to modern medicine. There is no need to present the evidence of the magnitude of the problem of mental illness in terms of social disability, economic loss, personal and family distress. Through countless professional journals and reports and through the daily press, popular magazines and books these matters have been brought to the attention of the general citizenry, as well as those engaged in health work, of most nations in western society, most notably in the United States.

As in all science, there are many chapters yet to be written and many, now written, that must and will continue to be rewritten. The breadth as well as the depth of the challenge is prodigious. Psychiatry is touched by and in turn touches the physical and biologic sciences, the social sciences and the humanities. It is not fortuitous that Jean Martin Charcot took for his motto the wise words of Terence, the Roman playwright, *"Homo sum: humani nihil a me alienum puto"* (I am a man and nothing that concerns a man do I deem a matter of indifference to me). I can think of no more proper inspiration for a psychiatrist; perhaps, one day, for all physicians.

But, what of the medical student who may read this chapter? What opportunities does he have in his medical school period to learn of the above, to meet intimately with those engaged in the pursuit of the objectives of modern psychiatry?

Ten years ago I noted that, with a few exceptions, psychiatry had little prestige value in the medical schools. Its assignment in medical school teaching had been with the care of the chronically mentally sick, obviously a matter of great concern to the nation's health, but just as obviously an aspect foreign to the central theme of medicine and distant from its central theater of operation in the university teaching hospital. Certain changes have occurred in the ten years that have elapsed. Although considerable unevenness continues to exist from school to school, an increasing number of the medical schools in the United States have established or are in the process of establishing departments of psychiatry comparable in some, if not all, respects to their fellow clinical departments in medicine, surgery, pediatrics and obstetrics.

In many schools the teaching of psychiatry continues to be responsible, most properly in my view, for the study, care, and treatment of the chronically mentally sick person, whether he be neurotic, psychotic, retarded or demented. However, this is no longer its exclusive concern. What are the reasons for this change? From my sample of experience it is uniquely American in its vigor and scope, quite different from what one observes in other parts of the world. But before we examine it, let us consider the medical student and the opportunities that he has before him in the medical school.

The Medical School.   Medicine is, indeed, a house of many mansions. Those who pursue its science and practice its art soon learn that they live and work in the world of things as well as in the world of persons. Medicine does and should call to it young men and women of diverse backgrounds, of different capacities, interests and abilities. Certainly, the creativity and curiosity of the gifted investigator, the parental generativity and judgment of the seasoned clinician, the capacity to deal objectively and yet compassionately with the pain, fear, shame and guilt of the sick person and his family, skills in administering things as well as men—these require qualities and experiences not commonly found in one person. I look, then, with misgiving on those who search for the stereotype candidate and I question the validity of current probability tests, such as medical vocational aptitude scales. The objective for which the prediction is made must be defined. Is it success in being admitted to a medical school, or mastery of the undergraduate course, or performance in graduate work in the laboratory or in the hospital, or in the eventual record of the established medical scientist and of the practicing physician?

In my view, the major purpose of the medical school is to help the student to prepare for whatever he eventually chooses to do in the fields of medical science and practice. Schools err when they adopt officially or unofficially ad hoc slogans such as, "It is our job to prepare our students for the general practice of medicine—or to become teachers—or investigators—or specialists—or administrators, etc." The primary responsibility of a school is to provide the scholarly atmosphere that will insure the soundest fundamental undergraduate medical education for each student. Whitehead's definition of the proper function of a university as being the imaginative acquisition of knowledge is no less true for the medical school than it is for the university as a whole. Each student, depending on his background, motivation, ability, and on the incentives and opportunities he seeks and finds, can hopefully become all that he is capable of becoming. He can then elect to pursue further the field of his choice. Each student should have ample opportunity to seek for and eventually to establish his own identity from his past heritage with its partial identifications and from the multiple models of scientists and physicians with whom he will be associated, as he will learn from them by example as well as by precept. It is hoped that this will be done consciously, cumulatively and intelligently without recourse to blind, neurotic choice and its subsequent restrictions.

A book like this, no matter how informative or how skillfully written, cannot, nor should it be intended to, serve as a substitute for the many years of thought and experience, perplexity, doubt and trial that determine individual choice and decision. At best, it can afford brief glimpses into special fields of interest. It may help, too, to correct the unevenness of experience that exists in all schools. Few schools offer equal opportunity for many, if not all, representatives of its faculties to meet intimately with students, to participate with them in their pursuits of knowledge and skill. This unevenness of opportunity within a faculty or from school to school, may be dependent upon many factors. Traditional beliefs and practices; the historical differences between disciplines in their acquisition of knowledge and skills; the success or failure in the application of new methods; changing patterns of morbidity and mortality; the emergence of faculty leaders with special concerns and influences and the degree of productive relatedness between the departments of a medical faculty; the amount of money available as well as facilities, laboratory and clinical, for research, teaching and service; the nature of the resolution of "town-gown" differences and of service responsibilities to the community; the geographic origins, vitality and scholarship of students and faculty; the operating relations between the medical school and its parent university—these as well as others—contribute to what emerges not once and for all time, but from time to time as the local signature, the central, idiosyncratic image of the medical school. These, too, determine the relative prestige position of the disciplines within the medical school.

My personal experience as a student and member of the faculties of six medical schools in the United States in the past twenty-five years has led me to inquire into the setting of the modern medical school. Many members of our faculties have not had the experience, now presented to their students, of considering systematically the many psychologic and social aspects of human behavior noted earlier. The situation is similar in some, but in not all respects, to the period of not much more than a generation ago when the medical faculties of that period grew up without benefit of systematic instruction in biochemistry, physiology and bacteriology. It is dissimilar in that in the earlier period, the pursuit of new and more precise knowledge in biochemistry, physiology and bacteriology bore a more direct, more linear relation to that which had been taught before. It also dealt with material which, for the most part, could be considered in "infra-human," certainly in impersonal terms. With psychiatry, if one is to be loyal to his material, one must grasp it as it permits, pursue it wherever it leads, and one must soon realize that he is dealing with matters of brain and mind, of mind and body, of human behavior, individual and group. The material, being more human, deals with man, not as an abstraction, but as a social organism in the theater of his moral and social values. When challenges and questions bear on matters, like those of infant and child care, sexual behavior, human aggres-

sion, socially deviant and irrational behavior, matters intimately interwoven in social and moral concepts, it is inevitable
that these meet with resistance, if not ridicule or attack. With
varying degrees of success and pain, most adults, including
members of the medical faculty, believe they have reached
judgments about these matters through their lifelong accumulation of experience in their private psychological worlds. It
is not easy and is often unpleasant to reconsider one's private
views unless there is adequate inner motivation to do so. But
this fact of omission, together with the various hegemonies of
faculty members who insist that there is really nothing new,
that, at best, it is common sense and that if they "had the
time" they would do as well, if not better, that which the
psychiatrist is trying to do—are these the full explanations?
I do not think so.

Perhaps with all beginnings there is much fumbling and
confusion, exaggerated therapeutic promises and premature
structuring of concepts. The psychiatrist should look to his
own house; his ignorance should not necessarily be compensated for by arrogant, long-winded jargon. If only the
strong can be gentle, I should think modern psychiatry is
strong enough to indicate however gently, but certainly
more clearly and succinctly, what it knows, what it thinks
it knows, and what it does not know. In all of science, a
theoretical concept exists only as a form of shorthand, an
attempt to explain in general terms, the relatedness or laws
between events previously thought to be unrelated. Survival
is dependent upon its usefulness in the pursuit of additional
knowledge, in its capacity to explain existing facts better
than any alternative. Allegiance to a theoretical concept,
experientially barren of new ideas, or to one which does not
explain existing facts better than another, is to my mind not
only dogma, but delusion. Eventually if psychiatry is to contribute to science it must remain loyal to its material and
adapt its methods appropriately to it. It must construct concepts that can be defended or refuted in scientific terms.
Science is cumulative. It cannot grow from declarations of

faith, no matter how piously or vigorously defended in terms of the complexity of the problem.

However uneven the opportunity for the medical student to share in the development of modern psychiatry, there is little question that today there are more opportunities in our medical schools than at any other time in their history. What has contributed to the greater interest and development of this subject in our American schools as compared with what I have observed in medical schools in the United Kingdom and on the European continent?

The American Scene. The mental health movement, uniquely vigorous in America, may perhaps be viewed in a broader sense, that is, of interest in the social sciences as a whole, including psychology. De Tocqueville, over a century ago, remarked on the pragmatic climate of the American scene; much of the philosophies of Pierce, James and Dewey have given further evidence of the accuracy of this penetrating observation so many years ago. Perhaps it is our naïveté, our optimism, our continuing belief in the modifiability of man. We believe that man is educable and through his capacity to deal in natural cause and effect sequences, is able to accumulate knowledge and apply it to solve his problems and to advance his welfare. While we appear to be much more interested in and informed about genic and ontogenetic forces as determinants of man's behavior than are the Soviet scientists I met, we are less prone than many of our European colleagues to look upon man's behavior as the inexorable unfolding of predetermined genic qualities, glancingly influenced by experience.

The mental health movement in itself has grown from the familiar and traditional Hippocratic form of reference, based upon the values of the relief of pain and suffering, of the reduction of social disability due to illness, of the preservation of life. Another source has come from the roots of Western humanism, concerned with the growth and development of the individual, with objectives of the full, mature, more creative life. A third source is that of the scientific discipline, by and of itself, its interest being primarily in the pursuit of knowledge for its own sake without regard to its immediate or eventual usefulness.

Our relative freedom from starvation and the ravages of catastrophic disease; our high standard of living; our greater freedom from tradition and perhaps greater ease in making changes; the speed and volume of communication, these, too, have been suggested as determinants of the vigor and growth of our interest in the social sciences, in psychology, and in mental health.

It is generally agreed that psychoanalytic psychology has had a significant impact on American psychiatry, certainly greater than on any other national medical scene of which I am aware. Its contributions to the concepts of the unconscious mind and of intrinsic biological drives, its exposition of the phenomena of transference and counter-transference in themselves are of basic and major importance in contributing to the core of what one day may become a basic science of human biology. It has evolved a conceptual scheme of mind or mental apparatus in genetic, dynamic, topographic, structural and economic terms. As a psychology of conflict it cannot serve as a general psychology, much less as a completely satisfactory or exclusive approach to a basic science of human biology conceived in social terms. Whether the limits of its instruments will permit it more fruitfully to pursue understanding of the human family, in health and sickness; of the relations between mind and brain, mind and body; whether it will one day become more useful and practical as a means of treatment are matters to be determined by further experience and more rigorously recorded evidence.

Although undoubtedly occurring in a setting of multiple determinants, the impact of psychoanalytic psychology has been a major factor in the increased interest in psychotherapy, particularly since the end of World War II. The accumulation of information and knowledge, the development of methods based upon certain principles has led in this century to a more structured approach. This, in turn, has attracted to it a greater number of psychiatrists who wish to engage in its practice; it has attracted, too, many patients who look eagerly to it for relief from their distress. Although there remain realistic difficulties together with the accumulated mutual tensions and sensitivities of the past fifty years, there is little doubt, from a comparative view of the United Kingdom and Europe, that we in the United States have reached a much more effective and hopefully more useful association between certain psychoanalytic institute faculties and the faculties of a number of university departments of psychiatry. While the dichotomy of the psychophobe and the biophobe are not unknown to us, few university departments follow slavishly an ideologic party line. In many American university departments there is the growth of broad eclectic interests in various bodies of knowledge and in the appointment of faculty members with different backgrounds, skills and interests. There are more university departments in which research with biochemical, neurophysiologic, psychologic, psychoanalytic, clinical psychologic, social, genetic and epidemiologic technics and knowledge take place in parallel, at times interrelated, and, occasionally, fruitful association. Here, too, parallel developments in the biologic sciences and in general medicine attest to common concern with more precise definitions of health and disease, with modern views of multiple causes and effects, of open rather than closed biologic systems, of dynamic steady states rather than fixed immutable equilibria.

The recognition by our Federal Government of the magnitude of social disability due to mental illness led our 79th Congress in 1946 to enact the National Mental Health Law. This provided the administrative medium through the United States Public Health Service for monies to be allocated for the education of psychologists, social case workers, psychiatrists and nurses; for the initiation and support of new researches in the broad field subsumed by mental health and illness; for grants in aid to state governments for certain types of new clinic facilities and mental health administrative organizations. In my view, the Federal program has been the single most useful and effective force in the growth and development of psychiatry in the United States in the past 14 years. Its influence has been felt primarily in the university departments but also at state, county, and local administrative levels where one may find new approaches in areas of prevention and rehabilitation as well as in hospital custody and treatment.

Parallel but independently there has been a rapid increase in the number of psychiatric units established in general hospitals, including some but not all university teaching hospitals. This, in itself, has reduced materially the isolation of the psychiatrist and his co-workers from the major theaters of medical teaching and research. In this new environment the psychiatrist has had to learn new methods to deal with human events quite different from those previously met by him in the sequestered mental hospital. University medical school departments of psychiatry have grown in number in the past fourteen years; in the number of full-time senior appointments within departments; in the area of clinical services for which they are responsible; in the range of research interests and activities within their departments, with their fellow clinical and pre-clinical departments in the medical school and with biology, psychology and the social sciences in the university as a whole; in the number and quality of candidates who apply for graduate career specialistic education; in the organization and devotion to their teaching programs, both undergraduate and graduate, and in their studies of epidemiology, prevention, etiology, diagnosis, treatment and rehabilitation.

With some exceptions, namely the recently established clinical center of the National Institute of Mental Health in Bethesda, several state hospital research units, private foundations and hospitals like the Menninger and Austen Riggs Foundations and the Chestnut Lodge Hospital and, of course, the psychoanalytic institutes, the principal areas for research and education increasingly have become the university departments based in units within the university teaching general hospitals. Here, they are engaged simultaneously in education at undergraduate and graduate levels; in research, participated in by students as well as senior faculty; and in clinical out-patient and in-patient services to their communities. The increase in the number and improvement in the quality of the candidates for career training in psychiatry is undoubtedly multiply determined. However, in our experience, we believe a significant factor to be that of the physical presence and active participating membership of the psychiatric faculty within the major teaching hospital scene. Through his teaching, his research activities, his day to day work in all the clinical areas of the hospital, the psychiatrist serves as a model, among other models, of the medical faculty. As indicated earlier, this enables each student, depending on his interest, aptitude, motivation and on the opportunity afforded him, to search for and eventually to establish his own identity from his past and from the multiple models of the faculty with whom he is associated.

If interested students should find little evidence of these developments in their medical schools or if their teachers appear to them to be uninformed or disinterested, I would suggest that they meet with students from other medical schools in order to compare their experiences. The recent establishment of summer student fellowship grants through the United States Public Health Service—National Institute of Mental Health for assignments in research and training offers many interesting opportunities for students to become acquainted with the work of departments of psychiatry in university medical school centers other than their own.

Internship.   Many students interested in pursuing the graduate study of psychiatry ask about the nature of the preparatory internship. In the official rules and regulations of the American Board of Psychiatry and Neurology, one finds only that there should be satisfactory completion of a year's internship approved by the Council on Medical Education and Hospitals of the American Medical Association in general medicine, general surgery, pediatrics or a rotating service. In the 1953 report on the internship in the United States, one will find references to certain aspects of clinical psychiatry during the internship. This modest but realistic statement reflected the existing limited opportunities in most first-year internships, straight, mixed or rotating, for any serious or significant psychiatric experience either as a direct assignment to a psychiatric service, or more importantly to liaison exercises and assignments between psychiatry and the other clinical disciplines. When students ask for my advice about the relative merits of the straight as compared with the rotating internship, I am unable to answer in the abstract. So much depends upon the student, his preparation, interest, and objective. Much depends, too, on the specific nature of the specific straight or specific rotating internship the student is considering. To assume that all straight internships are scholarly, afford continuity of patient care, intimate and continuous association with senior seasoned teachers, graduated responsibilities and the general pursuit of excellence; and that, in contrast, all rotating internships are vibrating, discontinuous, fragmented, elementary and essentially second class is, from my experience, not only mistaken, but absurd. In any instance, I advise my students to visit personally those hospitals in which they are interested and attempt to learn something of the faculty, their skill, experience and devotion to teaching; the physical facilities and operational policies of hospital and clinic as these relate to administrative ease or tedium, length of patient stay, follow up of patient, range of clinical material, age, sex, socio-economic group of patients, relations to the community health program; opportunity for graduated responsibilities in the study, care and treatment of the patient and his family, opportunities for the pursuit of new knowledge, library facilities, the measure of obligatory routine laboratory procedures, the relations between the clinical departments of the hospital, the history of the quality and destiny of house staff alumni and, most important of all, the over-all intellectual climate of the hospital, its eagerness or

indifference, restlessness or complacence in examining critically what it does and in planning imaginatively what it must
do tomorrow.

If the psychiatrist is to continue to be considered a physician, not a psychologist, it is necessary for the psychiatric
aspirant to search for and obtain, through his internship, a
full measure of continuing experience and knowledge in clinical medicine. So much the better if this can take place in a
teaching hospital where the basic approaches of psychiatry,
indispensable to all of medicine, those relating to the psychology and sociology of acute and chronic illness, convalescence, disability, surgical intervention, the patient-doctor relation are of common concern to all those who care for the
sick. Psychiatry as a special medical skill, I believe to be the
province of graduate training beyond the internship.

Psychiatric Residency. Psychiatry, among the various
medical specialties, was late in offering well-organized, systematic residency training programs. In 1936, 49 programs
offered 267 residences; in 1958, 268 programs reported a total
of 2,723 residents. As can be seen, this significant increase in
the number and also in the scope of teaching programs has
taken place within the past two decades. Informative historical
reviews of this development will be found in the report of the
Second Ithaca Conference (1952) and in recent studies of current and future trends in psychiatric residency training programs. The third edition (1960) of the *Descriptive Directory
of Psychiatric Training in the United States and Canada* con-
tains brief descriptions of psychiatric residency programs in
the United States and Canada.

The sources referred to will acquaint the student with certain historical landmarks of this development including the
educational interests of the American Psychiatric Association
and the National Association for Mental Health which led to
the establishment of the American Board of Psychiatry and
Neurology in 1934. One will also learn of the development
of the psychoanalytic institutes, begun in 1911 and of the
founding of the American Orthopsychiatric Association in

1924 to implement interest in child psychiatry. Several conferences in psychiatric education in 1933-1936 were valuable in assessing existing programs and in making constructive suggestions for the future. Military medical experience in World War II led a number of physicians to choose career training in psychiatry.

Today, few university and hospital centers appoint persons without personal visits of the candidates, as there appears to be general agreement that personal interviews are indispensable in any type of selection procedure. We urge our students, whether or not interviews are required, to visit the places they are considering and to learn as much as they can about those involved in it, at both junior and senior levels and, if possible, from the alumni of the program. We urge them, too, to learn what they can about the program from others in the medical center or hospital in which the program is located. Personal visits provide the candidate with opportunities to meet with members of the faculty, with the current peer group of residents, and to inspect the facilities, clinical, laboratory and library, and, hopefully, to learn something of the methods, substance, and objectives of the program. The faculties of some, certainly not all, teaching programs have become concerned with the selection of residents. This has come about because some centers have had sufficient numbers of applicants to choose among them and because of a genuine interest on the part of psychiatric teachers to search for adequate criteria for predicting a candidate's fitness for the field. Studies reported by the Group for the Advancement of Psychiatry's Committee on Medical Education, the Menninger Foundation Study and others reached the not-surprising conclusion that the ideal psychiatrist, like the ideal physician, eludes precise or adequate definition. Methods used include personal interviews, reports of past records in college, medical school, internship, and, less frequently, psychological tests. Letters of reference are usually requested from those with whom the candidate has worked intimately in school and hospital. Attention is directed to intelligence, physical and emo-

tional health, record of scholarly achievement, breadth of
interests, capacity for interpersonal relation, ability to perceive critically and honestly, successes or failures in life—in
his family, school, work, in marriage and parenthood; evidences of curiosity and originality and, what is usually subsumed under terms such as psychological mindedness, sensitivity, empathy, perceptiveness, intuition, interest in the
meaning and motivation of human behavior, that of self as
well as others. It means also the capacity for identification and,
as Eisendorfer indicates from his experience with psychoanalytic candidates, a passive capacity to listen and to understand. I would add, too, under this caption, the need for
resources sufficient to become able to deal with the pain
and distress of others without mobilizing unduly one's own
anxieties.

One should have, too, the appropriate interest and strength
to work in a field with many uncertainties and with tentative-
ness of knowledge. Andre Gide's remark may be relevant,
"He who explores the unknown must learn to walk alone."
While many of these qualities will be thought to be desirable
in all physicians, the psychiatrist, regardless of his many roles,
if he is to treat the sick, must be capable of drawing constantly
upon these from his repertory. One of the reasons offered as
explanation of the inability to define precisely the qualities
or personality characteristics of the ideal psychiatrist is that
of the wide range of activities now offered. Although these
are dependent upon the nature of university, medical school,
psychoanalytic institute, hospital, clinic and other facilities
in any community it becomes apparent that, as in legal education, the psychiatrist as he completes his formal preparation
for career work, and if his preparation is basic and thorough,
continues to have a wide array of activities from which to
choose for his life's work. It is impossible to delineate these
areas precisely, as in most instances today the practicing psychiatrist may be engaged in various combinations of the
following.

CAREER OPPORTUNITIES

General Practice of Psychiatry (Extramural). This usually consists of an office practice offering diagnostic, therapeutic, advisory and supportive services to patients and their families referred to the psychiatrist by his fellow physicians in the community. He may see children as well as adults, psychotic as well as neurotic patients and their families. He may have access to one or more private or public mental hospitals to which he may admit his patients and continue to be responsible in some way for their care and study. He may have part-time appointments in Veterans' Administration or state hospitals and clinics, in university or community clinics or hospitals. His therapeutic approaches may include the use of physical measures and drugs in addition to psychotherapy.

Special Practice of Psychiatry (Extramural). In addition to the above, others may devote a greater share of time in advisory or consultative services to children's and adult courts, to probation and police services, to public and Community Chest family and children's welfare, health and legal agencies; to other community services, including public educational measures in mental hygiene or preventive psychiatry. He may choose to restrict himself to a psychotherapeutic practice, attempting to deal more intensively in treatment with fewer patients over a longer period of time in what is called psychoanalytically oriented psychotherapy.

He may choose to obtain formal psychoanalytic training and establish himself as a practicing psychoanalyst, using this technic either exclusively for a limited number of patients or modifying it in some degree to care for a greater number. Here again he may or may not seek or obtain part-time appointments in clinical service, research and teaching in various teaching hospitals and clinics. He may be chosen to take part in administrative, educational and research activities of the psychoanalytic institute to which he is attached.

Psychiatrists have been invited to join small group medical practices made up of internists, surgeons, pediatricians, obstetricians which serve circumscribed population areas, urban and rural, throughout the nation.

Full-Time Hospital and Clinic Assignments (Intramural). The psychiatrist may choose to work as a clinical staff member of federal, state, county and community mental institutions and out-patient clinics. In some instances, in addition to his diagnostic and therapeutic work, he may take part in educational and research programs in his hospital and occasionally in other nearby institutions. Certain hospitals also permit a certain amount of extramural assignment for their full-time staffs in community affairs and in consultative practices.

Administrative, Educational, Supervisory. Traditional administrative posts in large mental hospitals have recently been stimulated by increasing interest in studies of the psychosocial setting of the hospital and has led to re-examination of the specific roles of the administrator as teacher and supervisor. Other types of administrative assignments are to be found in state mental health authorities. Federal agencies employing psychiatrists for administrative as well as other assignments include the Department of Defense, Veterans Administration, and the United States Public Health Service of the Department of Health, Education and Welfare.

New types of administrative assignments in the establishment of community mental health programs at city and county governmental levels are also being offered.

Administrative and educational posts dealing with problems of international health are to be found in the World Health Organization.

Military Assignments. In addition to the administrative assignments referred to earlier, the military psychiatrist may be engaged in preventive, educational, and evaluative assignments as well as in the care and study of individual patients. Opportunities for basic and applied research in scientific investigations relevant to military efforts are also available.

Student Health, Industry, Community Projects. Assignments of psychiatrists, either full- or part-time, to the staffs of elementary, secondary, collegiate, and professional schools offer opportunities for direct individual study and care of patients and for advisory and consultative services to principals, teachers, deans, dormitory supervisors in preventive and educational, as well as in diagnostic and therapeutic services. Similar opportunities are increasingly available in private industrial organizations and as advisors to those responsible for community projects such as civil defense; orientation programs for the police, clergy, welfare officers; housing projects, and neighborhood reclamation.

Educational and Research Assignments in Non-University Teaching Hospitals. In psychiatric units of general hospitals as well as in special mental hospitals, private and public, many psychiatrists in addition to teaching psychiatric residents are also engaged in teaching medical students and house officers from services other than psychiatry who may be assigned for varying periods to them. More often they share in the teaching of nursing staff and students, nursing assistants, the clergy, social case work and clinical psychology staff and students. They are also engaged in teaching those participating in patients' activities programs, students and staffs in occupational therapy, recreational therapy, music, drama, etc. In these hospitals and clinics they may also be involved in various basic and applied researches.

Non-University Research Institutions. The development of the Clinical Center of the National Institute of Mental Health in Bethesda has made possible opportunities at both junior and senior levels for research training and participation in basic (biochemical, neurophysiologic, psychologic, social) and in applied clinical and epidemiologic studies in the broad field subsumed by mental health and illness, child and adult and in many, if not all, clinical categories of neurotic, psychotic, and defective patients.

University Assignments. The operations of the university department of psychiatry with its teaching, research, and service obligations will be familiar to most students. As indicated earlier, more university departments have been established in psychiatric units intimately interwoven into the fabric of the central or principal teaching hospital of the university medical school. Thus the undergraduate teaching of medical students takes place in parallel with graduate teaching of psychiatric residents. In many places the residents assume graduated teaching responsibilities with medical students, nurses, and others. In these units emphasis has changed from major concern with diagnosis, commitments, and short-term stay to greater concern with more detailed studies of patients and their families, longer stay of patients, more intensive and active therapeutic programs to reduce the magnitude of chronic illness. The units together with their emergency admission divisions offer opportunities to study patients, young and old, from a broad socio-economic spectrum, acutely and chronically ill, including in instances patients and their families in acute normative emotional crises involving one or more members of the family. More intimate and active relations with community mental health programs permits the residents to learn at first hand of local and adjacent preventive, therapeutic, rehabilitative and custodial mental health facilities. The use of tutorial and other pedagogic supervisory technics assists the residents in their diagnostic and therapeutic responsibilities. Opportunities also exist in other departments of the medical school to take part in the teaching of medical students and house officers in the liaison programs between psychiatry and pediatrics, medicine, surgery, obstetrics and preventive medicine and with the teaching of students in the pursuit of researches with members of certain pre-clinical departments.

Research programs in university departments of psychiatry have been established in various associations with pre-clinical and clinical departments of the medical school and with psychology, biology, and the social sciences in the university as a whole. Psychiatry is attempting to create a new model, that of the clinical investigator, in addition to the traditional models of the psychotherapist and the administrator. The establishment of full-time research professorships and of senior and junior full-time research fellowships through private foundation funds, and increasingly through United States Public Health Service grants, attests to this. Up until recently, unlike the situation in medicine, the psychiatric resident has not had many opportunities to meet, much less learn of the methods and work of the scientific investigator in clinical psychiatry.

Psychiatrists have been invited to join the faculties of some schools of public health now engaged in preventive and educational pursuits as well as in epidemiologic and population studies of incidence and prevalence of mental disorder.

Child Psychiatry. The traditional opportunities in child-guidance clinics, institutions for retarded, psychotic and epileptic children and in courts and schools for delinquent children have now been extended into other areas. The work of the child psychiatrist in the university teaching hospital provides an opportunity for him to work intimately with pediatricians in well-baby clinics and in special clinics such as those concerned with cerebral palsy and other types of organic disease. Some of the university clinics have established nursery schools for healthy pre-school children as well as for those who are emotionally sick. Similarly, a number of universities have established intramural diagnostic and therapeutic services for school-age children. Special provisions for adolescents have also been made. A number of state hospitals as well as the clinical center of the United States Public Health Service are engaged in researches in and services for emotionally sick children. Children's hospitals have developed special units for emotionally sick children. In some communities residential treatment centers for long-term study and treatment of emotionally sick children provide additional opportunities for psychiatrists interested in and especially prepared to engage in intensive therapeutic study. Perhaps most important, the child psychiatrist working in a university teaching general hospital is playing an important part in teaching medical students and pediatric house officers on the children's floors and out-patient departments. Child psychiatrists continue to play important roles as advisors and consultants to community

children's agencies, schools, recreation and industrial programs, to the courts and institutions for the care, treatment,
and detention of delinquent children. Some child psychiatrists have become interested in the exciting new developments in biochemical researches in human genetics and in
learning problems as these relate to children with mental
defects.

This formidable but not exhaustive list of opportunities
that present themselves to the psychiatric careerist today cannot do full justice to the large number of combinations and
modifications of those mentioned. Small wonder, then, that
those who are responsible for the design and operation of
graduate teaching programs admit to perplexity as to what
should or should not, what can or cannot be included in the
graduate psychiatric curriculum.

GRADUATE CURRICULUM

Students may read with interest the section on curriculum
in the G.A.P. Committee's report, Chapter Three in the Second Ithaca Report; Boyd's comments on current and future
trends; and Gildea's chapter in the recently published "American Handbook of Psychiatry."

The American Board of Psychiatry and Neurology considers "desirable training" in the following terms. "The training for psychiatrists should include clinical work with psycho-
neurotic and psychotic patients, combined with the study of
basic psychiatric sciences, medical and social psychology, psychopathology, psychotherapy, and the physiological thera-
pies, including a basic knowledge of the form, function and
pertinent pathology of the nervous system. The training
should be supervised and guided by teachers competent to
develop skill and understanding in the utilization of such
basic knowledge in dealing with patients. Mere factual knowledge is not sufficient. This training period should include
instruction in the psychiatric aspects of general medical and
surgical conditions and the behavior disorders of children and
adolescents sufficient to develop practical ability to direct the

treatment of such conditions. It should also include collaborative work with social workers, clinical psychologists, courts and other social agencies. The training program of the candidate for certification in psychiatry should include sufficient training in neurology to enable him to recognize and to evaluate the evidences of organic and neurologic disease."

Admittedly, it is difficult to prepare statements of "desirable goals" without resorting to pious, subjunctive phrases, yet the statement does reflect the change that has taken place in graduate teaching in the past two decades. Serious attempts are being made by most persons responsible for designing and operating the pattern and objectives of programs to insure a full spectrum of clinical behavior of patients in terms of age, sex, socio-economic status, nature of distress (somatic, psychologic, social); to foster a climate of critical intellectual curiosity and interest among those who share in the study, care, and treatment of the sick, leading hopefully to the pursuit of new knowledge, and to the acquisition of the emotional security and knowledge of self adequate to insure compassionate but objective attitudes and skills in their therapeutic approaches with their patients. Obviously, inevitably, and in my view quite properly, the curriculum from program to program will vary considerably. Equally obvious is it that the curriculum in any one program should be changed whenever it is necessary to achieve new or old objectives more fully.

Arguments pro and con abound about the advantages and disadvantages of programs in mental hospitals, public or private, versus the psychiatric units in general hospitals; about brief block assignments versus long term assignments; about how many months should be devoted to psychiatric in-patient and out-patient services, medical and surgical assignments, psychiatric childrens' wards and neurology; of continuity in one center versus assignments in one or more affiliated or associated hospitals and clinics; to structured didactic exercises in neuroanatomy, neuropathology, psychodynamics, psychopathology, clinical psychology, sociology, etc., versus informal study of these matters starting from the resident's specific experiences with the patients for whom he is responsible.

Differences of opinion also exist about supervision, the responsibilities of the resident as physician, psychiatrist, psychotherapist, teacher. Some use tight tutorial supervision, others are less formal. Many are confused about the role of tutor or supervisor as pedagogue or as therapist to the resident. Some believe it best to provide formal compulsory courses in research methods, others believe that it is sufficient to provide an atmosphere conducive to the critical pursuit of new ideas in all members of the department and proceed from the individual interest rather than from required courses.

My own belief is that there will be and always should be these differences of opinion. They stem from tradition, experience, and prejudice. Many times they reflect unwittingly the broad or circumscribed interests of the faculty in teaching, service and research; they may betray the abundance or limitation of space, funds, number of faculty, service needs, and relations with other departments in the teaching hospital.

In the past two decades there has emerged a fairly uniform pattern, perhaps influenced to some degree by the requirements for certification of the American Board of Psychiatry and Neurology. (Admission to the examination for certification in psychiatry requires a total of five calendar years of training and experience, three years of which must be specialized training satisfactorily completed in approved training centers, plus two years of experience.)

My personal view is that the goal should not necessarily become that of uniformity but rather of continuing attempts to examine critically what is being done and to make changes whenever and wherever necessary to improve what we now do.

Earlier mention was made of the inclusion of neurology. In this matter, interested students will read with profit the papers presented by Yakovlev and Alpers. I believe that clinical neurologic experience is indispensable to the training of a psychiatrist. I am less convinced of the success of routine, didactic courses in neuroanatomy, pathology, chemistry and physiology other than for "refresher" purposes. If the resident exhibits spontaneous and sustained interest in these matters, every opportunity should be afforded him to pursue his inclination from his special point of departure.

As mentioned earlier, a more complex and controversial matter is that of formal psychoanalytic training during the psychiatric residency. Those interested will be rewarded by reading the report, recently published, by Lewin and Ross of their survey of psychoanalytic education in the United States. In it the reader will find a vast fund of information about the historical, pedagogical, administrative and psychological aspects of psychoanalytic education.

That there is considerable interest among residents in obtaining such education is undeniable as is the fact that many so inclined appear to be motivated because of interests in psychotherapy. There are others, however, who seek such education not for the traditional role of the practicing psychoanalytic therapist but look to it for its eventual usefulness in the general or special practices of psychiatry, as teachers and in the pursuit of research. I believe there are real differences in the methods and objectives between psychiatric residency programs and those established in psychoanalytic institutes. Historically, the psychiatric residency programs are in transition. The impact of psychoanalytic psychology, in terms of its contributions to the understanding of the dynamic unconscious mind, of transference and countertransference in the therapeutic setting, have become intimately interwoven into the fabric of history taking, of interviewing, as well as of formal therapeutic approach. They constitute the essence of the attempts to understand the content of irrational human behavior. The university programs are trying to incorporate these significant contributions into the broader, more comprehensive experience and responsibility of the clinical psychiatrist, in his multiple diagnostic, advisory and therapeutic roles. In and out of the universities, investigators are also attempting to test more precisely and record more rigorously the primary data obtained from psychoanalytic method. This has raised the question of the appropriateness of psychoanalytic institute training for those who may not wish to become traditional psychoanalytic therapists.

Parallel with this is the dilemma in which the psychoanalytic institutes find themselves in terms of defending the purity of their identity or of participating in the general integration and adaptation of method and substance into the broader areas of general psychology and of clinical psychiatry. Whether phobic or not, eclectic deterioration is a fate most institute faculties fear.

Alexander has written thoughtfully and imaginatively about the distinctions between psychotherapy and psychoanalysis. Kubie has for many years suggested a basic reorganization of psychiatric education, imaginatively conceived but impractical.

While I do not minimize the difficulties and complexities of the current scene, I believe that our American pragmatism may eventually find a solution. Although most institutes require at least a year's work in psychiatry at application and the completion of three years of psychiatry by the time of graduation from the institute, many of them choose as their candidates those with most psychiatric experience. In our university we do not permit residents to engage in didactic psychoanalysis during the first two years and only infrequently in their third year. We have found over the past eighteen years in two university settings (Cincinnati and Rochester) that the first-year resident is more than fully occupied in his assignment, with its new challenges and problems. To add to this, the experience of personal analysis has neither benefited the resident nor his patients.

In general, in advising our students who seek graduate training in psychiatry, we return again to the general principles alluded to earlier which applied to his experiences in the medical school and in the internship.

If the setting provides for a community of scholars, who through common interests and experience look critically, perceptively, and imaginatively at their data; if the range of clinical behavior is sufficiently broad; if there are multiple models of scholars, old and young, with different backgrounds, experiences, and interests; if there are provisions for graduated and continuous responsibilities with adequate supervision in the study, care and treatment of the sick; if the library is alive, and if there are opportunities, if one wishes, to explore the unknown and to walk alone;—if the resident in turn is sufficiently intelligent, reasonably healthy, industrious and well-motivated, he will usually find himself well prepared to choose that which he wishes to do among the great number of opportunities before him. Our experience leads us to emphasize the need for a broad, thorough, fundamental experience in clinical psychiatry from which point the resident may choose further, consciously and wisely, what he wishes to do.

There is much to do. Collegiate preparation for medicine in the future may permit more students to obtain a sound liberal educational background.

Tomorrow's medical schools, unless the classes become too large, may achieve, through the efforts of their faculties, a clearer understanding among those who share in common the venture of teaching medical students. It is quite likely that there will be a gradual improvement in the teaching of psychiatry in the medical schools. What will happen to the internship of tomorrow, among other things, will be dependent upon service needs but in general will continue to insure more educational opportunities.

Liaison teaching and research programs between psychiatry and the other clinical disciplines may be established in additional centers depending upon special facilities and interests and, most important, upon the recruitment and firm support of persons courageous enough to explore mutant roles between disciplines.

One may predict that more psychiatric units will be established in general, including university teaching hospitals. This will necessitate effecting intimate and productive working relations between them and special hospitals for mentally sick patients.

In the graduate psychiatric residency programs, I believe there will be a movement toward expansion of clinical service and teaching in emergency first aid centers in addition to traditional clinic and hospital services. I would hope that teaching programs would become more intimately intertwined with the activities of those engaged in basic and applied research in the many areas of neurochemistry and physiology, psychology, and sociology relevant to the furtherance of scholarship in clinical psychiatry. Much, of course, is yet to be learned about the appropriateness and results of our therapeutic efforts. More is to be done in prevention.

As in all health sciences, the greatest good will come from that knowledge, which, if applied will lead to prevention. I know of no role in our modern society better suited to apply sound principles of mental health to the patient and his family than that of the family doctor if he should survive in our country. He can be and often is close to the patient and his family, and if alert and informed may help to guide his patients properly toward those measures, which, if initiated early, may prevent the development of psychologic illness. In other ways, the point is applicable to all physicians regardless of their field of work. It is for this reason that I believe one of the most important responsibilities of modern psychiatry to be the education of medical students. If tomorrow's physicians can acquire the attitude and knowledge appropriate to understanding their patients' problems, permitting them to identify distress early, advise with thought and caution, treat that which is within their skills to do and to refer intelligently to others that which needs special or technical skills not possessed by them, much will be gained.

The history of medicine, including psychiatry, is a window through which one may look out upon mankind. Through its window, psychiatry can teach us how man, over centuries of written records, perceived his fellow men thought to be possessed, mad or sick. One may learn, too, of the cyclic changes in attitudes and how these were determined by economic, political and religious factors in settings of ignorance, fear and want as well as by the body empiric of clinical information and knowledge. Few but vigorous were the voices of courageous humanists and physicians who insisted on naturalistic approaches to that which appeared magical and supernatural to the others.

Santayana's caution, "Those who cannot remember the past are condemned to repeat it" may have a special meaning to psychiatry. Has its history been circular, and is there less evidence of the historical spiral of progress than in other fields of medicine? Whether true or not it should lead the student to examine more thoroughly the record of the past to understand better where we are and where we may go.

As a psychiatrist, I never fail to be astonished by the daily opportunities to grow in knowledge and wisdom. It has been my good fortune to serve in a number of medical schools, hospitals and clinics as teacher, clinician, administrator and clinical investigator. I am most grateful to those who teach me—my patients, my students and my colleagues. Psychiatry affords many occasions to acquire and pursue specialistic, circumscribed interests and skills in the multiple areas of its relevance; however, in it, if one chooses, one may also retain that which is indeed rare in our day, particularly in modern medicine, namely, a generalistic approach to the nature of human behavior. It is the most personal, the most human of the medical sciences. Terence's maxim will be as appropriate tomorrow as it is today and as it was to Charcot a century ago. "I am a man and nothing that concerns a man do I deem a matter of indifference to me."

BIBLIOGRAPHY

Romano, J.: Basic orientation and education of the medical student, J.A.M.A. *143*:409-412, 1950.

Romano, J., ed.: Adaptation, Ithaca, N. Y., Cornell Univ. Press, 1949.

Romano, J.: Psychiatry in undergraduate medical education, Bull. Menninger Clinic *9*:34-40, 1945.

Romano, J.: The Physician as a Comprehensive Human Biologist in Education for Professional Responsibility, Pittsburgh, Carnegie Press, 1948.

Engel, G. L.: Unified concept of health and disease, Perspectives in Biology and Medicine III, pp. 459-485, 1960.

Guillain, G.: J. M. Charcot. Edited and translated by Pearce Bailey. New York, Hoeber, 1959.

Witenberg, E. G., Rioch, J. M., and Mazer, M.: The Interpersonal and Cultural Approaches, vol. II, Chapter 70, pp. 1417-1433, The American Handbook of Psychiatry, New York, Basic Books, 1959.

Sanford, F. H.: Paper presented at National Health Forum, Cincinnati, Ohio, March 22, 1957. Joint Commission on Mental Illness and Health.

Report of the Advisory Committee on Interns to the Council on Medical Education in Hospitals of the American Medical Association, J.A.M.A. *151*:499-510, 1953.

Revision of the Essentials of an Approved Internship, J.A.M.A. *151*:579-585, February 14, 1953.

The Psychiatrist, His Training and Development, Report of the 1952 Ithaca Conference, American Psychiatric Association, Washington, 1953.

Group for the Advancement of Psychiatry, Trends and Issues in Psychiatric Residency Programs, Report No. 31, March, 1955, Publications Office, 3617 West Sixth Avenue, Topeka, Kansas.

Boyd, D. A., Jr.: Current and future trends in psychiatric residency training, J. Med. Education *33*:341-351, 1958.

Holt, R. R., and Luborsky, L.: Personality Pattern of Psychiatrists, New York, Basic Books, 1958.

A Descriptive Directory of Psychiatric Training in the United States and Canada, American Psychiatric Association, Washington 9, D. C., 1960.

Ebaugh, F. G., and Rymer, C. A.: Psychiatry in Medical Education, New York, The Commonwealth Fund, 1942.

Eisendorfer, A.: The selection of candidates applying for psychoanalytic training, Psychoanalyt. Quart. *28*:374-378, 1959.

Gildea, E. F.: Teaching of Psychiatry to Residents, American Handbook of Psychiatry, vol. II, pp. 1935-1947, New York, Basic Books, 1959.

Rosenbaum, M.: Problems in supervision of psychiatric residents in psychotherapy, A.M.A. Arch. Neurol. & Psychiat. *69*:43-48, 1953.

Romano, J.: Discussion of Brosin, H. W.: On discovery and experiment in psychiatry, Am. J. Psychiat. *111*:561-575, 1955.

Lewin, B. D., and Ross, H.: Psychoanalytic Education in the United States, New York, Norton, 1960.

Alexander, F.: Psychoanalysis and Psychotherapy, New York, Norton, 1956.

Kubie, L. S.: Need for a new discipline in the medical profession, A.M.A. Arch. Neurol. & Psychiat. *78*:283-293, 1957.

Severinghaus, A. E., Carman, H. J., and Cadbury, W. E., Jr.: Preparation for Medical Education in the Liberal Arts College, New York, McGraw-Hill, 1953.

Deitrick, J. E., and Berson, R. C.: Medical Schools in the United States at Mid-Century, New York, McGraw-Hill, 1953.

Psychiatry and Medical Education. Report of the 1951 Ithaca Conference, Washington, American Psychiatric Association, 1952.

Levine, M., and Lederer, H. D.: Teaching of Psychiatry in Medical Schools, American Handbook of Psychiatry, vol. II, pp. 1923-1934, New York, Basic Books, 1959.

Romano, J., and Engel, G. L.: Teaching experiences in general hospitals, Am. J. Orthopsychiatry *17*:602-604, 1947.

An Outline for a Curriculum for Teaching Psychiatry in Medical Schools, Prepared by the Committee on Medical Education of the American Psychiatric Association, J. Med. Education *31*:115-128, 1956.

Romano, J.: Conference on Psychiatric Education, J. Med. Education *27*:167-175, 1952.

Curran, J. A.: Internships and residencies, historical backgrounds and current trends, J. Med. Education *34*:873-884, 1959.

Wilson, K. M., Donovan, J. C., and Romano, J.: An experiment in the teaching of obstetrics and gynecology at the graduate level, Am. J. Obst. *66*:654-662, 1953.

Engel, G. L., Greene, W. A., Jr., Reichsman, F., Schmale, A., and Ashenburg, N.: A graduate and undergraduate teaching program on the psychological aspects of medicine, J. Med. Education *32*:859-870, 1957.

Ackerknecht. E. J.: A Short History of Psychiatry, New York, Hafner, 1959.

Deutsch, A.: The Mentally Ill in America, Garden City, N. Y., Doubleday, 1937.

Bromberg, W.: Man Above Humanity, Philadelphia, Lippincott, 1954.

Zilboorg, G., and Henry, G. W.: A History of Medical Psychology, New York, Norton, 1941.

Freud, S.: An Autobiographical Study, London, Hogarth, 1936.

Jones, E.: The Life and Work of Sigmund Freud, Vol. I (1953), II (1955), III (1957), New York, Basic Books.

8

Surgery

Some men are born surgeons. J. M. T. Finney, a surgical giant in the illustrious history of the Johns Hopkins, never had a doubt about studying medicine nor a qualm about becoming a surgeon. Lord Lister, the father of antiseptic surgery, made up his mind to be a surgeon at the age of thirteen. His choice was instinctive and spontaneous because none of his close relatives or family friends were doctors and none of the Listers had been professional men of any kind. Other men are attracted early in life to medicine but at first think they may not have the temperament of a surgeon. Samuel Gross of Philadelphia, founder of the American Surgical Association, and in many ways the father of modern American surgery was so sensitive that he fainted the first time he saw blood drawn, and throughout his life hated to watch an operation. Many, perhaps most men, reach the decision to be a surgeon gradually. The choice is finally determined by the influence of a particular person—a family doctor, a teacher or a friend. Sometimes chance settles the matter.

Harvey Cushing, who became the Moseley professor of surgery at Harvard and the world's greatest brain surgeon, wanted to be a biochemist when he was in college. Later, chance may have made him a surgeon. When Cushing was finishing his house officership at the Massachusetts General Hospital in Boston, he was determined to get additional experience at the new Johns Hopkins University Hospital in Baltimore. He wrote to W. S. Thayer whom he had once met inquiring about the opportunities in the department of medicine under Professor William Osler. When Thayer, who was deeply involved in research in malaria, failed to reply, Cushing wrote to Halsted, the professor of surgery. Halsted answered promptly and ultimately offered Cushing an appointment as an assistant resident in surgery. Early in his career, however, Cushing became an intimate friend of Professor Osler who exerted a profound influence on him throughout his life. Had he started with Osler as a resident in medicine it seems certain that surgery would have been deprived of his genius. If Thayer's preoccupation with malarial research is weighed in this episode it can be argued that the meteoric development of neurosurgery by Harvey Cushing was incident to the bite of the mosquito.

In just such ways great lives are molded, but most men cannot wait for the bite of the mosquito. They feel obliged to give their future considerable thought. Some unfortunates become so concerned with the future that they fail in the present. The best advice in this respect is to trust in the future, forget the past, and give all one has to the vital and important now. There is only one thing to guard against in selecting a special field of medicine and particularly is this true of surgery—do not make the final decision too soon.

Often a young man interested in surgery is told to "come up to the hospital and see an operation" or "get a job working in the operating room and see how you like it." This is well intended but poor advice. It can do no good and it may do harm. At its best it is an unprofitable disbursement of time for a man whose life will be spent in the operating room. At its worst it is comparable to pushing a child of three off a diving board to see if he takes to swimming. He may, but it is more likely that after such an experience even a potential Olympic swimmer would prefer croquet or bowling on the lawn. So it is with surgery. Watching an operation is a foolish first approach to its science and art. An able but sensitive person can be turned away because he sees it as a spectacle rather than a single decisive act in the total care of a sick man.

"The practice of surgery," writes Francis D. Moore, the present Moseley professor of surgery at Harvard, "is the assumption of *complete responsibility* for the welfare of the patient suffering from injury and wounds, local infections, tumors, and a large fraction of various pathologic processes and anomalies which are localized to the organs of the body." No comprehension of this immense prospect, nor any inkling as to whether one is fitted for the responsibilities involved, can be obtained by a premature visit to the floor of a hospital operating theater.

How then, should one approach the important decision of selecting surgery as a career? First, give it no serious thought before entering medical school. It is enough to make a firm decision to study medicine. It is fundamental that the prospective surgeon be attracted to medicine as a whole, because he must become a good doctor if he is to be a good surgeon. Even though there may be leanings toward surgery, or as in Lister's case, a determination to be a surgeon, one should give the matter no heed and waste no time in putting emotions to a premature test.

Once launched on the study of medicine, there is no more salutary way of exploring fields of special interest than the reading of the lives of the great physicians, surgeons and investigators of the past. Read the lives of John Hunter, Pasteur, Lister, Osler, Samuel Gross, Welch, Halsted, Cushing, Moynihan, the Mayos—there is scarcely any end to the list. Select a few including Cushing's life of Osler and read deeply. If the going gets heavy, relax with "Arrowsmith," or the "Citadel," or "Of Human Bondage." Add to the above a generous sampling of the essays of Osler, Thayer, Moynihan, Cushing, and Ogilvie and by the end of the second year in medical school, the time will be ripe to give serious consideration to a career in surgery. Indeed, it will follow naturally upon the student's introduction to the care of the surgical patient, for responsibility for the care of the patient is the essence of surgery.

Historically and actually there are certain differences between medicine and surgery. Medicine had its early beginnings in witchcraft and in religion. The physician was a priest who dispelled the evil spirits of disease.

On the other hand surgery sprang from injury and war. There were no mysteries about it. The surgeon was a warrior who displayed a special talent for binding the wounds of his companions. This distinction between the physician, who was a priest, and the surgeon, who was a "dresser of wounds," can be found in the Egyptian papyrus, in Homer and in the Bible. From the beginning, therefore, surgery has been more practical than medicine and the results of surgical treatment have been more immediate and apparent. The distinction has not always been complimentary to surgery. In the thirteenth century, surgery was looked upon as a degrading craft beneath the dignity of the physicians who were cultured men belonging to the upper classes. Surgeons were identified with the barbers. Despite important contributions to the care of wounds by Henri de Mondeville, de Chauliac, and Ambroise Paré, the barber-surgeons flourished throughout Europe, an uneducated, untrained band engaged in shaving, hair cutting, blood-letting, and operating. Meanwhile, the cornerstones of surgery were being quarried by Leonardo da Vinci, Versalius, and William Harvey—but the laying of the stones and the building of the edifice were still far away.

The student must read for himself of the men and the contributions that have made surgery a science and an art rather than a craft. To read of John Hunter and the experimental method, of John Collins Warren and anesthesia, of Lister and antisepsis, and of Halsted and surgical technic, is but a beginning. The growth of surgery as a science raised on the foundations of anatomy, physiology, pathology, and biochemistry, is wonderfully portrayed in the history of the Harvard Medical School and the life of J. Collins Warren, son of John Collins Warren. (See "To Work in the Vineyard of Surgery," edited by E. D. Churchill.)

Today, surgery is an applied science as well as a healing art, and the surgeon bears an enormous responsibility for the care of the sick. He must be well-grounded in anatomy, pathology, bacteriology, chemistry, and physiology. He must be a good physician with an intimate knowledge of the natural history and clinical manifestations of injury and disease. Finally, he must recognize that surgery, which in the beginning was separated from medicine and the priesthood, has, pari passu with its growth as a science, become closer to medicine and more of a ministry. This role is thrust upon the surgeon as well as upon his medical colleagues by the anxious patient who wants his doctor not just as an engineer or a scientist but as a friend and a sympathetic minister. Thus, there are three aspects to the practice of surgery—the knowledge of it as an applied science, the application of it as a form of human biology, and the practice of it as a healing art.

What manner of man is attracted to this profession? Are there still sharp distinctions between physician and surgeon? All manner of men and not a few women enter surgery, and all manner of men and women become accomplished and distinguished surgeons. The complexities of modern medicine have drawn the surgeon and the physician together, increasing their mutual respect and making the "team-approach" to the seriously ill patient a daily necessity. Yet, the responsibilities of physician and surgeon remain distinct. One or the other must be in charge of the patient. When an operation is in prospect or has been performed, the surgeon cannot delegate his responsibilities to his medical colleague. And just as the responsibilities of physician and surgeon remain distinct, so in a general way, their personalities differ. Sir Heneage Ogilvie, one of Britain's great men of surgery, has written delightfully and pointedly on this subject. He believes that the surgeon is more apt to have been an athlete, a football player, or a yachtsman, and the physician a debater, an editor of the school paper, or if he takes to a sport, it is apt to be golf. While all will not agree with this view, the student is urged to read Ogilvie's "A Surgeon's Life," "Religio Chirurgi," and "The Training of a Surgeon."

The differences between physician and surgeon tend to be overemphasized. The best surgeons would make excellent internists, and the best internists, if chance had so influenced their choice, would be capable surgeons. There are two qualities, however, that are essential for the surgeon; without them he is gravely handicapped, and yet might be a capable physician or investigator. First is a reasonable degree of manual facility. Little needs to be said about this because, by and large, the hopelessly clumsy are not attracted to surgery. Occasionally, however, a very superior mind is possessed of mediocre hands. In such circumstances, the individual enters a surgical career with a permanent handicap. In medicine, no such barrier exists.

The second quality without which even the most capable individuals cannot be accomplished surgeons is the power to make a decision promptly and decisively on the basis of evidence that at times must be incomplete. There are many men, scholars, investigators and intellectual leaders who do not have this quality. They see a problem so clearly and so all inclusively that the inadequacy of the evidence prevents them from arriving at a decision. In military life, such men make staff officers. They are superb at planning. They can see all possibilities and anticipate every eventuality. Faced with a particular crisis, however, they want all the data before they can act. As field commanders they are lost. The field commander may not be as brilliant, he may not even be as well versed in the theories of military tactics, but he possesses this singular type of judgment, the invaluable gift of acting with precision on the basis of incomplete evidence and being right. He also has the perception and skill to change his mind as the situation changes. He can bail himself out of a wrong decision before it is too late. This particular kind of judgment is obvious in the leadership of Lee, Jackson and Grant. Its almost complete absence in McClellan and Meade, both brilliant staff officers, nearly cost the North the war. Lincoln said of McClellan, "He has 'the slows.' He is an admirable engineer but he seems to have a special talent for a stationary engine."

A sharp distinction must be made here between this special

kind of judgment and the making of "snap judgments." A snap judgment is made without using all the evidence available. The men who make snap judgments are often well informed and self assured. They can be very useful so long as major responsibility does not fall on their shoulders. Under pressure they jump to conclusions, become obstinate and lose perception. Commander Queeg, victim of the mutiny on the "Caine" was an extreme example. General Pope's actions in the campaign against Lee and Jackson from Cedar Mountain to the disaster at Second Bull Run is an actual and more typical case. Such men cannot lead.

So it is with surgery. A man with "the slows" will miss the "golden moment" when an operation can be safely performed in the course of a critical illness. One who makes snap judgments will rush in too soon or unnecessarily. The accomplished surgeon must know all he can about his patient and the injury or disease in question. In consultation with his colleague, the physician, he must review all aspects of the case. He must be familiar with all possible eventualities and he can leave no stone unturned in preparing himself and his patient for an operation. He cannot make a hasty or snap judgment, but human biology is so complex and the manifestations of injury and disease so varied that with all the data available, the surgeon is repeatedly faced not with a certainty but only with a balanced probability. On this basis, he must act to operate or not to operate and a life may hang in the balance.

The quality of judgment is highly desirable in the physician but the very nature of most medical ailments permits more prolonged and often continuing study before any crucial decision is reached. Often, the decision can be deferred until more information is available or the general progress of the disease becomes manifest. Ogilvie has compared the physician's task to that of a golfer. He strives to play a particular course as skillfully and carefully as possible. He may get a low score or a high score, but he will complete the game in the end. "The ground will not split beneath his feet nor will the game change suddenly from golf to bull fighting." The surgeon is constantly being called on for decisions based on his estimate of the probable course of events rather than on predictable developments. To quote Ogilvie, "He is like the skipper of an ocean-going yacht. He knows the port he must make, but he cannot foresee the course of the journey. He must be guided as he goes by changes of wind and weather." To return to the military analogy, the surgeon is like a field commander who knows his objective but cannot predict what moves the enemy may make. The whole plan of an operation may have to be altered on a second's notice because of some unforeseen complication. One cannot wait to obtain all the information before making a decision. Like the field commander resisting the shock of an enemy attack, a decision must be made before waiting for intelligence reports that may be days in coming. The battle is the pay-off and the surgeon is always at the front.

Because he must so often act positively, the surgeon is more accountable than the physician. This is why responsibility is so repeatedly emphasized as the essence of good surgical practice. "Surgery is total responsibility," as Francis D. Moore has said. "The guiding circumstance of the surgeon's life is personal responsibility" Sir Heneage Ogilvie wrote in 1948, "This adds to the interest that surgery possesses and to the *responsibility* which is entailed on those who practice it" according to Sir Benjamin Brodie (1846). The American Board of Surgery, whose task is to certify that a surgeon is qualified to practice his specialty, places "senior responsibility" as the essential feature of the education of the surgeon.

The development of "senior responsibility" takes time. Elliott Cutler, who succeeded Harvey Cushing at Harvard always said "it takes seven years to make a surgeon." The minimum time required by the American Board of Surgery is four years after the completion of an internship. Many men elect a longer period. Experience in the major subspecialties of surgery is a part of the education of the surgeon. A particular interest in vascular or cancer work may require an additional year or two. Time in the research laboratory is a golden experience. In fact the young man who goes directly into practice from a four-year residency is still in need of experience. He is qualified but not seasoned. But no matter how long he trains, the surgeon's education is never complete. His is a life of continuing self-education and growth. He must run hard to keep abreast of progress. If he fails to do so he will fall behind and soon will be unable to meet his responsibility as a surgeon.

Responsibility can weigh heavily at times. Every surgeon of experience knows long nights and dark days. Sometimes, as Dr. John Mulholland said in his presidential address before the American Surgical Association, the surgeon wonders why he did not choose some less exacting vocation. "He wishes he were a clerk and could be home in bed with no responsibility." But no issue in surgery can be avoided. With worthier motive than Macbeth, the surgeon must repeatedly "screw his courage to the sticking-place." But then comes the dawn with a period of triumph. The difficult and trying operation proves a complete success. All his patients are well. Suddenly the affection of his patients, the admiration of his juniors and the respect of his colleagues become amazingly obvious and meaningful. He is on top of the world—until tomorrow's crisis. No profession is so fraught with emotional turbulence. Each surgeon reacts in his own way. Some are visibly strained by the difficult moments and heartened by the periods of serenity and success. Others take trial and triumph with a steely calm easily mistaken for coldness or indifference by those who do not know them well.

While a good measure of equanimity and imperturbability are invaluable assets to the surgeon, a few great surgeons in the past have worn their emotions on their sleeve. The great John Homans of Harvard used to punctuate an operation by bursts of song, "A wandering minstrel I, a thing of shreds and patches, of ballads, songs, and snatches and dreamy lullaby." During one particularly long procedure he got through most of the Mikado. Other surgeons, equally distinguished, made every operation an ordeal for their assistants. The trend is away from this today. The danger of spreading infection by unnecessary talking makes silence in the operating theater essential, in the best traditions of Halsted and Cushing. There is no place in modern surgery for the extreme emotional outbursts that were characteristic of some great surgeons of the past. If a man cannot control himself under the daily pressures of surgery, he is well advised to consider some less demanding branch of medicine.

Two other virtues, one essential and the other most becoming to the surgeon, are intellectual honesty and humility. Because so many decisions rest on a probability rather than a certainty, every untoward result following an operation must be critically reviewed. A thoughtful reappraisal in the light of subsequent events may indicate some other course of action in a similar situation in the future. Intellectual honesty is, therefore, essential to the continued growth of the individual surgeon. Experience accumulated from such reappraisals constitutes the basis for much of surgical progress. Those who cannot face up to the facts and draw lessons from their mistakes are doomed to a life of self deception. They have no place in medicine. In surgery their work is lethal.

Humility graces any man. It is especially good for the surgeon. It makes a frank appraisal of his mistakes easier and it leads to a sympathetic understanding of the difficulties of his fellow surgeons. Most of all, it helps him to keep his accomplishments in proper perspective, for although the responsibilities of surgery are great, the rewards are even greater. Despite the strain and pressures, most operations today are successful. Moreover, in the mind of the patient every operation, whether it is followed by complications or not, is a positive act of salvation so that while he loves his physician he is prone to worship his surgeon. Surrounded by this adulation, the surgeon of wide experience is easily led to a favorable opinion of himself. After all, Aesculapius was only a successful practitioner until Zeus struck him with a thunder bolt and made him the God of medicine. So as the surgeon climbs his own Olympian height, be he professor in a medical school, a leader in a large private clinic or a distinguished practitioner in a small community, it is easy for him to become lost in the clouds. A bit of humility will remind him that his feet are clay, the mountain illusory and the clouds more foggy than ethereal.

Intellectual honesty, the gift of judgment and a keen sense of responsibility are essential attributes of the surgeon. Equanimity and humility grace his work. The fulfillment of his career, however, like that of his brother, the physician, requires hard **work,** and **charity,** for "the law of the higher life is only fulfilled by love." The bonds of friendship are never forged so well as when men are joined in a common struggle. War, which threatens man's annihilation, unites him in deepest brotherhood. War is hard and so, in its way is surgery. But when it is hardest it binds men of good will together, patient and doctor, physician and surgeon, and surgeon and surgeon. For the accomplished surgeon these bonds of understanding friendship are the true rewards of his profession.

How well the surgeons of today and yesterday have met their obligations a young man must determine for himself. In so doing, perhaps he will be moved to become a surgeon of tomorrow and labor in the same vineyard.

CARROLL B. LARSON, M.D.
Professor of Orthopedic Surgery at the University of Iowa

9

Orthopedic Surgery

Orthopedic surgery is that branch of the art especially concerned with the preservation and restoration of function of
the skeletal system, its articulations and its associated structures. Early Greek texts bear testimony with amazing clarity
to the antiquity of this venerable branch of surgery in the
discussion of scoliosis, clubfoot, fractures and dislocations,
and chronic bone and joint infections. The word "orthopédie" was synthesized by Nicholas Andry, in 1741, from the
Greek roots "orthos" (straight) and "paidion" (child), when
he submitted the proposition that the prevention of deformed
adults lay in the development of straight children. The term
in its anglicized form "Orthopaedia" appears in the first
English edition of Andry's book, published in London in
1743.

Orthopedic surgery became in fact, if not in organization,
a marked specialty in the eighteenth century when the first
hospital devoted exclusively to orthopedic cases, and even
maintaining its own brace shop, was opened by Venel at
Orbe, Switzerland. Because of the extensive application of
braces to many different human deformities, orthopedic surgeons were for many years looked upon as brace-makers.
Gradually, however, with the advent of antisepsis and the
x-ray, surgical correction became possible. Successful bone
transplantation and grafting then developed from the experimental work of MacEwen in Glasgow. In 1826 John Ray

Barton of Philadelphia produced a pseudarthrosis or false joint by the operation of osteotomy. This opened a new era for arthroplasties, which were applied in rapid progression to many joints of the body, and were the forerunners of present-day technics for making new joints. In 1847, in Italy, bone-shortening and bone-lengthening operations were attempted, and in 1911 Albee and Hibbs of New York City carried out the first successful spinal fusions.

The common orthopedic problems are likely to be recognized by any recent graduate of a medical college. Many of these he learns as accompaniments of a disease or condition studied as part of a course in internal medicine, neurology, or pediatrics—such as the deformity of a joint as part of rheumatoid arthritis, a drop-foot as the result of a neurologic disorder, or a congenital dislocation of the hip as one of many other deformities to be found in pediatric patients.

The medical schools of our country average a total of sixty hours assigned to orthopedic surgery out of the four-year curriculum; hence, it would be unreasonable to expect a recent graduate to know the details of management of each of these problems. By the same token, the idea of orthopedic surgery as a career seldom occurs to the student during undergraduate days unless he has come to know it by some prior experience.

The internship is the time when the new doctor deals directly with the varied problems in medicine and it is a stimulating period, for he finds that principles and theories learned in school suddenly become responsibilities and realities. It is likely that while he is working in the surgical wards or the emergency room, a particular case will provide the challenge that turns his interest to orthopedic surgery. Let us say that he is faced with a problem of a fractured hip in an elderly woman who is known to have diabetes. He had learned a few facts about diabetes and a few facts about a fractured hip but the combination of the two poses a new problem. Which should be treated first and how is one condition related to the other? The patient is in pain and needs an x-ray and an evaluation of her diabetes. It is possible that the diabetes is out of control because of the pain, and an operation on the hip to control the pain may further aggravate the diabetes.

The arrival of the orthopedic consultant helps to put each factor in its proper relation to the other. An intravenous solution of glucose fortified with insulin is immediately injected as a continuous drip into the patient's vein, the leg kept comfortable by manual traction while the patient is transported to the x-ray room for adequate x-ray pictures, and soon she is back in her room where, under local anesthesia, a small metal pin is drilled through the bone below the knee. Through this device traction on the leg is maintained. With the patient comfortable in bed it is possible to evaluate the diabetes and bring it under control. Days pass and the orthopedic surgeon adjusts the traction from time to time to bring the fractured bones into alignment, using portable x-rays as a guide.

The intern reviews his anatomy so that he may better understand the mechanics of the situation. Thus, in this one case, the intern finds the orthopedic surgeon not only well versed in the anatomy of the extremities and the mechanism of muscles acting across joints but also in the complications presented by the diabetes and the psychological stresses of the situation.

Orthopedic surgery thus may come to intrigue him as a possible career, as he realizes that here is a specialty requiring an extremely broad scope of medical knowledge and making direct application of a basic science such as anatomy.

The minimum standards of training for the field are set by the American Board of Orthopedic Surgery. This is a self-incorporated body of orthopedic surgeons representing the American Academy of Orthopedic Surgeons, the American Orthopedic Association, and the Orthopedic Section of the American Medical Association. It works in liaison with the Council on Hospitals of the American Medical Association, which inspects training centers to see that they meet prescribed standards. The organization is similar to that of many other medical specialties. For a prescribed training in orthopedic surgery the Board requires a degree in medicine from an approved school, an internship, one year of surgical residency training and three years spent in orthopedic surgery in an approved residency program. On completion of these requirements, the aspirant is entitled to apply to the Board for examination and if successful in passing Parts I and II, he becomes Board-qualified. The qualification guarantees the maintenance of high standards of orthopedic care. Anyone holding a state license to practice medicine has a right to practice orthopedic surgery whether or not he is a diplomate of the Board. An advantage of securing Board-qualification is that it is often a requisite for appointment to hospital staffs including Veterans Administration hospitals and those associated with the Federal Crippled Children's Bureau. In addition, Board-qualified orthopedists are usually called as consultants in industrial and medical-legal problems.

Since its incorporation in 1934, the American Board has already qualified over 3,000 orthopedic surgeons, most of whom are now in active practice. Twenty-six hundred of these are members of the American Academy of Orthopaedic Surgeons, which is the largest national orthopedic medical organization. This means that there is a ratio of one orthopedic surgeon to approximately each hundred and fifty thousand population.

Perhaps the greatest impetus to a public understanding of orthopedic surgery came about as a result of World War II. Sixty per cent of the medical problems of the Armed Forces during the war were cared for by orthopedic surgeons, having resulted from wounds involving the extremities and spine for the most part, but also including all common types of bone and joint disability such as flat-feet, torn cartilages in the knee, backaches, recurring dislocations of the shoulder, strains and sprains and amputations, and the fitting of artificial limbs.

Because the field of human biomechanics has expanded

rapidly, many orthopedic surgeons today have gone on to further specialization. It is thus that the specialty has come to include such fields as hip surgery, hand surgery, congenital deformities and muscle transplantations, a device of specialization that has encouraged continued progress.

In 1954, the Orthopedic Research Society was founded by those members engaged in investigative work in the basic areas pertinent to the field, such as the electron microscopic pattern of bone structure, the metabolism of calcium and bone formation, the enzyme systems of cartilage, and studies on metallic implants in the body. It is obvious that the opportunities in orthopedic surgery are ever increasing, providing ample areas not only for practice of the specialty but for careers in academic medicine as well as untold possibilities for research.

The responsibilities of an orthopedic surgeon are those common to any physician in any specialty. First of all, he must adhere to the code of ethics that applies to all physicians. As a specialist he fits into the medical family as a consultant and is not in competition with his colleagues in any other area. He must utilize his knowledge to help those who come to consult him and he must give advice with prudence. He must join and serve national and local medical organizations, take part in providing disability examinations, and serve as expert witness to aid the courts in attaining justice in medical-legal matters. Above all, he must maintain an educational continuum through the current literature, attending instructional courses and so preserving an open mind toward any change that shows promise of improved therapy.

Orthopedic surgery, like all branches of medicine, offers a life of eminent satisfaction. This, as with any medical career stems from the relation of doctor to patient. Within this intimate relation, the physician is able to counsel wisely, for through the problems that he has had to meet he has learned to know himself, as was counseled by the philosophers.

Benjamin Tenney, M.D.

*Clinical Professor of Obstetrics and Gynecology
at Harvard Medical School*

10

Obstetrics and Gynecology

Mention of obstetrics and gynecology brings to mind the deliveries of infants, and hysterectomies. While admittedly important, these procedures involve only a small part of the practice of this combined specialty. Obstetrics and gynecology actually involve the practice of medicine as much as that of surgery. Of the patients seen in the office of the gynecologist, only 10 to 15 per cent are hospitalized for surgery, a large proportion requiring medical treatment. In the pregnant woman, such complications as heart disease, diabetes, and renal disease are frequently a greater problem and constitute more of a challenge than the actual delivery. Certain other medical problems are the result of a pregnancy itself, the physiologic changes of which affect the diagnosis and treatment of many medical complications.

Major surgery in this field is as varied and interesting as in any surgical specialty, for in some ways it is more closely related to physiology and pathology than it is in many other areas. Some of the extensive surgery for cancer, for example, involves prolonged training and a high degree of skill. Competence in abdominal surgery is necessary, and vaginal and plastic surgery require, in addition, a thorough training in a multitude of procedures.

Endocrinology is a major and important part of obstetrics and gynecology, for the reproductive tract is particularly sensitive to endocrine control, and hormone imbalance is a common problem. This special knowledge applies particularly to infertility and involves not only endocrine but mechanical and psychic factors, as well as actual disease. This problem offers unlimited possibilities for investigation.

Embryology and the physiology of the growth and development of the fetus also constitute an important field of endeavor, and the fetal environment, which is so important to the mental and physiologic health of the newborn, offers promising opportunities for investigation.

Cancer of the reproductive tract is one of the major problems of gynecology, involving preventive medicine, as in the proper care of the cervix following delivery. Early diagnosis by various methods of screening is most important, and routine pelvic examinations are indicated as women approach the cancer age. Treatment involves a thorough understanding of radiation therapy and special training in surgery for cancer. The uterus is one of the favorable sites for investigation of cancer and for the improvement of therapy.

Because of its close association with the reproductive tract, the urinary tract also is involved in many gynecologic problems and a sound knowledge of urology is essential in this specialty.

Whereas, up to recent times, obstetrics and gynecology have lagged behind in laboratory research, this deficiency is being rapidly overcome, many young men are entering into research in this field and much excellent work is resulting. The clinician, biochemist, physicist, endocrinologist and pathologist have united in many clinics for the purpose of solving basic problems. Research funds are accumulating, and many opportunities are now available for young men to follow their special interests.

One cannot draw any definite line between obstetrics and gynecology for the two actually constitute one field dealing with reproduction and with the disorders and diseases of the reproductive tract. There is a single purpose and that is to preserve the function of reproduction where possible, at the same time preserving a woman's health in the face of damage or disease.

It is vital, therefore, that the physician entering this specialty receive a broad training in it since its various areas cannot be separated. However, with this basic understanding, one can devote his energy to the specialty as a whole or to any selected area he may choose.

History. Among all primitive peoples, childbirth and the menstrual pattern have been closely associated with religious and other taboos, with the involvement of much mysticism and magic. However, the basic problem of this function in relation to the survival of the race has been well recognized, and from the dawn of history records are available showing the importance attached to reproduction. From ancient Egypt, Babylonia, India, and China come written evidence of various forms of obstetric practice. Whereas anatomy and physiology in the modern sense had not been explored, there is evidence of efforts to aid the safe delivery of the infant. The problem was largely left in the hands of women although there are references to medical aid in the presence of complications. Since the great majority of pregnant women will deliver themselves safely, if there is no interference with the normal process of labor, we assume that most children were born safely, and certainly the maternal mortality was not sufficient to interfere with the increase of the human race.

With the development of Greek civilization and its interest in medicine, there was considerable speculation concerning obstetrics and gynecology. In the "Corpus Hippocraticum" there are several treatises on this subject and much discussion of female physiology and pregnancy. Many of the ideas derived from earlier civilizations were blended with the observations of the Hippocratic group.

In Rome one first hears of male obstetricians and it was there that the "lex regia" was enforced. This involved an abdominal section to remove the infant from all women who died during labor, before burial of the mother was permitted.

Soranus, who flourished between 98 and 138 A.D. wrote a text on the diseases of women. In addition to anatomy, he discussed such subjects as version, contraception, prolapse of the uterus, inflammation and the use of pessaries and even mentioned inversion of the uterus from traction on the cord. In the sixth century, there were reports on malpositions of the uterus, breast abscess, carcinoma and eclampsia.

For the next thousand years, there was little change or advance in the field, relatively untrained midwives delivering the human race until, in the sixteenth and seventeenth centuries, textbooks on obstetrics and gynecology began to appear on the European continent. Some of these were translated into English. The revival of podalic version and the development of obstetric forceps were the major events, most complications of delivery being handled by podalic version. A host of forceps were developed of which the most famous were devised and used in France by the Chamberlen family, members of which migrated to England with the invention. The secret was kept in the family for some time, but by the end of the seventeenth century it was widely known.

Cesarean section had early become a familiar procedure. In 1500, Jacob Nufer performed this operation on his wife, who survived, and several sections were reported in the sixteenth century, notably fifteen successful cases by Rousset. There was no suture of the uterus or ligation of vessels, but the abdominal wall was closed by various technics.

In gynecology, extrauterine pregnancy was discussed as well as rupture of the uterus, vesicovaginal fistulas were recognized and some attempt at repair was made. Ovariectomy was mentioned but there is a question as to whether it was performed.

In the eighteenth century, the emphasis that Smellie and Baudelocque placed on pelvic measurement and anatomy did much to change obstetrics from a clumsy effort to a more skillful art, and the obstetric forceps was adapted to the pelvic curve. France was a center of teaching at this period, although the development of the Rotunda in Dublin had a marked influence in favor of conservative obstetrics. This institution was strongly opposed to cesarean section.

The development of large maternity hospitals caused widespread epidemics of fatal puerperal fever, the control of which was achieved only gradually. Semmelweis made one of the notable early contributions to understanding it and Oliver Wendell Holmes and others suspected its contagious nature. Pasteur finally demonstrated the etiologic agent.

The work of Lister in developing antiseptic surgery and the later advent of asepsis did much to advance obstetrics and gynecology, modern gynecologic surgery having been made possible by asepsis and its scope having been extended by blood transfusion and antibiotics.

As we look back, we must realize the degree to which modern knowledge and technics have contributed to the development of this field. Much that we believe to be true will prove to be wrong in the years to come, for it is only by constant trial and observation that we can slowly correct our ignorance.

Importance to Society. Nothing can be more important for the future of the human race than the birth of normal infants. Unfortunately, at the present time, institutions are full of physically and mentally defective children, many of whom were damaged during pregnancy or delivery. Some of the harm could have been avoided with proper obstetric care, and as our understanding of fetal physiology and environment increases, such injuries will more and more become preventable. In addition to accidents and avoidable trauma during delivery, the effects of such diseases as diabetes and nephritis occurring are being better understood, and fetal damage is decreasing.

Prematurity presents an increasingly difficult problem. Because of the increased knowledge and skill of the pediatrician more and smaller babies are being salvaged than ever before. Unfortunately, the younger and smaller the premature infant the more susceptible it is to mental and physical defects and many of these children fail to develop normally. Whereas this is a pediatric problem, the obstetrician has a basic responsibility to give the infant the best possible chance in life by a safe and nontraumatic delivery. The conduct of labor, the selection of analgesics and anesthetic agents and the type of delivery are all important factors in effecting this result.

The obstetrician has an equally grave responsibility in regard to the prenatal care and delivery of infants whose mothers are under his care. He must in as far as possible take care that no disease, no problem of malnutrition or other complication of pregnancy injures the infant during its intra-uterine life. Anoxia and other fetal depression must be avoided during labor, and delivery must be accomplished with the least possible trauma to the infant. Poor prenatal supervision, improper conduct of labor and poorly performed deliveries may all cause permanent damage to the baby.

The health of the mother is of paramount importance, for in our society she is the most important factor in the later care and development of her children. Any illness or chronic disability that affects her will affect adversely their proper adjustment to life. It is the aim of good obstetrics to have the patient in as good or better health following the birth of an infant than she was before, and good obstetric care will bring the great majority of women safely through pregnancy with no residual impairment of health.

The recognition and early treatment of such physical damage as may occur during childbirth will in most cases restore the patient to full health, and proper postpartum care will also greatly reduce the danger of malignant disease in later years.

Throughout her life's span, woman is subject to disorders of the reproductive organs. Many such disorders are related to childbirth and many are not. Again, early diagnosis and treatment, medical or surgical, will usually preserve health and happiness.

Personal Satisfaction. The specialty of obstetrics and gynecology offers much in the way of satisfaction and reward to the physician who is drawn to this field, but it is not the place for one who is seeking an easy and regular existence. It is a demanding specialty both physically and psychologically. One must have the desire to serve, a liking for patients, and a detached, mature approach. A certain sacrifice of personal desires and pleasures to patient needs is necessary.

Obstetrics and gynecology is more like general practice than are most other specialties. Not only does it cover a wide field of medicine and surgery but the relation of the doctor to his patients and often to their families is that of physician, friend and adviser. The good specialist must keep abreast of developments in both medicine and surgery for he may well encounter almost any medical complication during the course of a patient's pregnancy. Surgical problems may arise during parturition and he may be involved in the medical and surgical disorders of the patient's future life. In spite of advanced education and business careers, the production of children and the raising of a family remain the most important goal of the average woman's life. To the doctor who has safely delivered her of a healthy child, she has a deep sense of loyalty and gratitude; she believes that he is the best doctor of them all.

A patient, and often the husband, having been seen frequently by the obstetrician during one or more pregnancies, a strong friendship and a deep trust often develops between the physician and the family. He becomes their adviser in many diverse problems and he is often called on in medical and other emergencies for personal help or direction. It is a pleasant relation that tends to continue through life.

It is well known that in any hospital, the obstetric floor is the happiest in the hospital with not only the patients but also the doctors and nurses sharing in the never ending joy of childbirth. The visits to the new mother with her healthy baby are a continuing pleasure to the obstetrician, who enjoys true satisfaction in having fulfilled a deep responsibility. Even in the occasional tragedy where all has not turned out well, the sympathy and understanding for the distraught young mother can bring an even deeper understanding and a firmer bond between patient and physician.

There is no specialty in which personal integrity and honesty is more important than in obstetrics and gynecology. Not only is the personal relation of the physician to his patients involved, but he is the only one who can possibly know whether he has done good work or not. The public yardstick of whether a mother and baby have left the hospital alive, or a patient has successfully recovered from an operation is of no value in considering the quality of work performed. A baby that is mentally or physically damaged due to poor obstetrics is a permanent tragedy. A mother may become an invalid for life due to poor judgment or procedure. In surgery, one must carefully consider whether the operation was really indicated and properly executed. Was the childbearing function unnecessarily destroyed or was the patient's normal endocrine health unwisely upset? It is only the physician himself who is in the position to give an honest answer to these questions. If he is honest and has erred, he will admit it and suffer. He will learn by the error and try not to repeat his mistake. If he will not face the truth within himself, he will not learn, and will repeat his mistakes. He cannot fool himself for long, however, and his life will be a tormented existence.

   Training.   Since obstetrics and gynecology represent such a broad field, one should have a preparatory general training before entering into residency training for this specialty. Considering the economics involved, there has to be a limit to the number of years that most young men can spend in preparation. The addition of two years of military service for many doctors makes the time factor even more acute. The minimum requirement to qualify for the American Board of Obstetrics and Gynecology is one year of internship and three years of residency training. However, it is a wise investment to allow five years rather than four to prepare for this specialty. A year in medicine followed by a year in general surgery is an excellent preparation for residency training, with a good two-year rotating internship probably equally good. A basic knowledge of medicine is essential and whereas one year of general surgery does not make a general surgeon it provides the opportunity to obtain an experience with differential diagnosis and a knowledge of general surgical pathology. One should be able to recognize gross pathology that may be unexpectedly encountered on entering the abdomen, in addition to which the gynecologist should be able to handle such bowel surgery as may be indicated in an emergency situation. The addition of experience with urology in a rotating service is most helpful, although a reasonable knowledge of urology is required in most residency training programs.

Some training programs in obstetrics and gynecology require two years of general surgery before an applicant is accepted. This is based on the belief that such experience is necessary for the future performance of major gynecologic surgery. The differences between the philosophy and requirements of the heads of training programs make it advisable for the young doctor to investigate such departments well in advance, and plan his preparation accordingly.

In those cases where training programs accept a candidate after one year's internship, a rotating service is the most generally recommended.

A few clinics have developed five-year training programs in obstetrics and gynecology. Some of these include the internship year and others do not. Whereas I personally believe that an internship in any specialty is inadvisable, this overspecialization is compensated for in many general hospitals by rotating the intern through the other departments. The five-year residency training program is usually designed to develop teachers and investigators, rather than practitioners. This has its advantages as well as its disadvantages. If there is a pyramid system, certain men are dropped at the end of three years with possibly inadequate training, though they are qualified for the American Board. The ones that survive the full five years are usually exceptionally well trained.

It is necessary to warn young men against accepting appointments in one- or two-year training programs. In the first place, the American Board frowns on a training at several different hospitals as there is usually much repetition and a man may end up with three years of first- or second-year experience. An even more important factor is the negligible chance of entering a good training program above the first-year level. Either the resident has to accept an inferior third-year appointment, or, as has happened not infrequently, he has to start all over at the first-year level on a three-year program.

In investigating a program, a candidate should ascertain the amount of service material that is available for residency training. In small clinics with a predominance of private patients there is often not enough material for sufficient experience in the specialty. While it is true that there are not enough good training programs to take care of all applicants, a well qualified applicant should be able to obtain a good training in this specialty.

Training programs in the military service are not primarily designed to supply practitioners for civilian practice, and in general they are not available to reserve officers but are limited to doctors in the regular service. Under any conditions, one is obligated for a year's service for each year of training. It has become a definite policy of the armed forces that an officer who has specialty training shall work in that specialty and not be assigned to other duty.

The training programs in obstetrics and gynecology in the armed forces and the caliber of work performed is the equal of that in good civilian institutions, for the training hospitals of the armed services are situated in or near civilian medical centers and make abundant use of civilian teachers for training and consultation. Each department is headed by a member of the American Board and there is usually an additional diplomate on the staff. The departments have the best and most modern equipment and all patients are available for residency training and can be studied and treated, within reason, without regard to expense. The patient load in the dependents' service is ample for the number of residents assigned.

One can practice excellent obstetrics and gynecology in the Service and under present conditions the net financial return, including retirement pay, does not differ greatly from that of private practice. One is definitely a member of

the military establishment, however, and should not undertake such a career unless one's goals and ambitions are compatible with military life.

Teaching vs. Practice. For the minority of young men
who are interested in an academic career following their
training in obstetrics and gynecology, there are many opportunities in this field. To attempt such a career, however, the
young doctor must have a real interest in teaching and investigation. In addition, he must be willing to receive less
financial return than that offered by private practice. Teaching is moreover a difficult art and requires much time and
application. A natural instinct for teaching is of great assistance and most men can discover during a residency training
whether they enjoy their teaching assignments or not.
Research, clinical or laboratory, is a must for an academic
career and so much emphasis has been placed on it in the
medical schools that many men, totally unqualified, are lured
into this field. One must have a constant curiosity, a detached
approach, intellectual integrity, and a tendency to carry on
in the face of repeated disappointments. Such a combination
of qualities is not common. Many investigators are poor
teachers and yet have to carry a heavy teaching load. In fact,
the emphasis on research has become so great that teaching
has suffered as a consequence.

The young man with proper qualifications will have no
difficulty in finding a position in the academic world. This
may involve additional years of training in special fields but
he will be well subsidized during this period and once
properly prepared he will have a choice of several medical
schools and appointments. His field of special interest will be
largely of his own choosing.

The majority of men in training will enter private practice,
however, which is as it should be. The status of the private
practitioner in society and in his profession is as great and
often greater than that of his academic brother, in addition
to which the personal satisfaction from the care of private
patients is often greater than that derived from institutional

medicine. In most medical centers, moreover, there is an opportunity for the practitioner to take part in the clinical teaching of medical students.

The irregular hours and night work frequently discourage young men from entering obstetrics. In our changing society, however, the public is becoming accustomed to practice by associates or groups and most obstetricians are entering practice under these conditions. Such arrangements allow for regular nights and weekends off and satisfactory vacations. Too large groups can destroy the proper relation of doctor to patient, but two or three associates, who know their patients in common, can actually give them better care by having one of them always available and all of them getting sufficient rest and relaxation. In addition, they have the time and energy to keep up with the literature and take such postgraduate courses as they choose.

Whereas it is true that there is not a clear cut line between the practitioner and those in academic life, the line is becoming sharper each year. Nevertheless, many men in academic life still take care of private patients and many practitioners teach, although private practice and teaching do interfere with each other. Medical schools are relying more and more on the full-time staff, and the practitioner is doing less and less teaching with the result that the young doctor must set his course in one direction or the other early in his career.

J. Hartwell Harrison, M.D.

*Clinical Professor of Genito-Urinary Surgery
at Harvard Medical School*

11

Urology

Urology has developed as a specialty in the field of surgery
during the last seventy-five years because of the necessity for
special instruments, technics and facilities to manage the
disorders of the genito-urinary system. On the other hand
genitourinary surgery is one of the oldest specialties in the
art of surgery and has really only in the last two decades been
removed slightly from general surgery and placed in the
sphere of the urologist. The history of urology, therefore, is
a segment of the evolution of surgery itself as well as the
history of those physicians who were especially interested in
the treatment of urinary infections and the complications
thereof, and who, in years gone by were often not really
surgeons at all.

Circumcision, one of the earliest operations, has been
performed since 4000 B.C. or thereabouts. Other urologic
operations were undertaken by itinerant barber surgeons
whose major activity was "cutting for the stone," a maneuver
attended by high mortality, high morbidity and great suffering for the patient and in all probability for the surgeon as
well. Therefore these gentlemen, such as Frère Jacques, were
forced to keep on the move because of the severe complications of hemorrhage and sepsis.

The hollow tube has long been prominent in surgery as
shown in the Egyptian writings of 3440 B.C. when such

instruments of tin and brass were used as catheters. Later the
Greeks, Romans and Chinese employed similar instruments.
Erasistratus (310-250 B.C.) treated strictures of the urethra
with an S-shaped catheter. The ruins of Pompeii, buried by
volcanic eruptions in 79 A.D., have yielded a number of
metal catheters, sounds and probes. Galen (131-210 A.D.)
also described an S-shaped catheter and the Arabians in 980-
1037 A.D., led by Avicenna, adapted Galen's teachings to
their own use and developed the first flexible catheter. No
further improvements of significance occurred until the 18th
century when a flexible tube made of a spiral of flat silver
covered with cloth was introduced. Benjamin Franklin invented a flexible catheter in Philadelphia in 1760.

In France Leroy D'Etoiles in 1822, Civiale in 1824, and
Heurteloup in 1824, introduced a lithotrite and had very
bitter disputes as to priority of its invention. Henry Jacob
Bigelow of Boston later introduced the surgical procedure
of litholapaxy, or the crushing of a stone in the bladder, and
invented the renowned Bigelow evacuator and lithotrite for
treating vesical calculi. In 1860 August Nélaton following
the discovery of methods of processing rubber in the 19th
century made an improved and valuable flexible rubber
catheter. Twenty years ago the availability of soft latex permitted the development, by Fred Foley, of a self-retaining
type of catheter with a balloon, which has been so useful in
alleviating the discomfort of urinary retention.

In 1845 Maisonneuve produced the flexible filiform bougie
which could be passed beyond even a very narrow stricture
of the urethra and to which a larger instrument could be
attached for the purpose of dilatation. All of these weapons
were "blind" and during the 19th century the search for a
means of seeing into the urethra and bladder was begun.
Bozzini and Segalis were among those prominent in such
efforts. The latter invented a speculum lit by two candles
which was held at the mouth of the instrument by the
observer's hands and thus gave light enough for him to
cauterize granulations of the urethra, and even to examine
a stone in a female child's bladder. Desormeaux in 1853 used

a direct endoscope with an oil light for illumination. Max Nitze of Germany in 1885 perfected the cystoscope using the incandescent light of Edison which, for the first time, made possible accurate visualization of the urethra and bladder. Kelley of Johns Hopkins was the first to succeed in catheterizing the ureter in the female, but it was Joachim Albarron in 1897 who perfected the ureteral catheter and became the father of modern cystoscopic diagnosis. Sir Astley Cooper of London (1768-1841), a pupil of John Hunter, published in 1830 his classic book *"Diseases of the Testis."* One of the greatest of the French urologic teachers was Felix Guyon (1831-1920) who was famous for his lectures on disease of the bladder and prostate. He perfected Bigelow's litholapaxy while serving on the Paris faculty.

Konrad Roentgen announced his discovery of x-ray in 1897 and Volcker and von Lichtenberg shortly discovered that roentgenograms of the urinary bladder could be produced by instilling colloidal silver solution into that organ to serve as a contrast medium. They found that sometimes the material would enter the ureter and renal pelvis as well. Later they made deliberate attempts to fill the renal pelvis by means of the ureteral catheters of Albarran. This resulted in successful pyelograms in 1906. Rowntree and his associates at the Mayo Clinic found that the intravenous injection of 200 cc. of 15 per cent sodium iodide would faintly outline the renal pelvis and bladder. Professor Arthur Binz who succeeded Dr. Paul Ehrlich developed uroselectan while searching for a better treatment for syphilis than salvarsan. When injected intravenously this radiopaque compound was selectively excreted by the kidneys. In 1930 von Lichtenberg and Swick used uroselectan to develop the modern technic of excretory urography.

Aortography and renal arteriography were introduced by dos Santos in 1929. Subsequently Doss, Nelson and Parke-Smith improved arteriography for the demonstration of various pathologic lesions of the kidney and renal vessels especially those associated with hypertension.

Advances in the technic of laminography have led to better

diagnostic measures in regard to the adrenal as well as to the kidney. Dr. George Cahill in 1935 made the first report on the use of perinephric insufflation of air to determine the presence of a suspected adrenal tumor. The insufflation of retroperitoneal gases via the presacral route was initiated by Ruiz-Rivas as an aid in outlining tumors of the retroperitoneal space.

Of equal importance with the advance of x-ray and instrumental technics have been advances in physiology and biochemistry, which have led to better understanding of renal failure and metabolic disorders involving the various glands of internal secretion, especially the adrenal cortex and medulla. Advances in the field of environmental sepsis, bacteriology, antibiotics, the application of principles of asepsis in the management of the catheter, as well as in surgical technics, have resulted in vast improvement in the diagnosis and treatment of disorders of the genitourinary system.

It is apparent that the specialty of urology has come into being as a field of surgery because of the necessity for the development of particular diagnostic and therapeutic technics in the management of diseases of the genitourinary system. It is essential that the urologist have a background in general surgery and equally essential that every general surgeon have basic training in urology. Progress in the management of genitourinary diseases in the past century has been made as a result of the progress in general surgery, anesthesia, the basic sciences, instrumental technology, biological chemistry, bacteriology and radiology. Prior to the beginning of the 20th century and during its first decade the urologist was primarily a physician who treated venereal disease and other types of urinary infection as well as disorders of the skin. Diagnostic urology was in its infancy and urologic surgery was still largely done by the general surgeon. As instruments and technics improved, the time consuming nature of the diagnostic procedures demanded that one doing urology should be willing to devote himself to this endeavor in order to maintain efficiency and to continue to progress in the field. One could no longer practice general surgery and have time also to carry out the practice of urology.

Urologic surgery today is found at the crossroads of general surgery and general medicine because it is deeply involved in each. It has a strong appeal for the surgeon who enjoys establishing his observations by means of actual measurement. In the laboratory of the cystoscopic department he uses the microscope daily in his studies of cytology and bacteriology of the urinary sediment. Colony counts are made on the cultures of the urine by the bacteriologist and exacting sensitivity studies are made for the specific therapy of the infection that is present. He carries out physiologic measurements of renal function of the two kidneys together and separately. He makes his own roentgenograms, develops them immediately, and is able immediately to make decisions for the next step in diagnosis and treatment of his patients. Physiologic measurements of the function of the musculature of the urinary bladder are made by means of the cystometrogram. A thorough understanding of the autonomic as well as of the central nervous system and their control over the genitourinary organs is of basic importance and is applied regularly.

The investigation of the patient always demands a complete history and physical examination. Urinalysis, hematology, the chemistry of the blood with special emphasis on nitrogen and electrolyte balance, are all of major importance in genitourinary disease. In the roentgenographic investigation of the patient the plain film of the abdomen and chest serve as the basic controls in x-ray. This may be followed by an excretory urogram, which is a serial and physiologic demonstration of the collecting system of the upper, middle and lower urinary tract following the injection of a non-toxic organic iodide preparation which has a selective affinity for the kidneys and is promptly excreted by them. Thanks to the development of the urethroscope and cystoscope, visualization of the urethra and bladder can be carried out accurately to supplement information gained by urethrogram and cystogram. The location of the source of bleeding or infection in

the urinary tract may be accurately accomplished by means
of the cystoscope and the ureteral catheter. Further sharp
delineation of the ureters and renal pelves can be accomplished by the introduction of opaque medium through a
ureteral catheter to make a retrograde pyelogram. These diagnostic procedures are usually carried out under local anesthesia in the adult and under general anesthesia in children.
Operative cystoscopic work is always done under general anesthesia. The ureteral catheter as a therapeutic instrument
serves to relieve the kidney blocked by a stone in the ureter,
or by an intrinsic or extrinsic tumor obstructing the ureter.
Similarly the urethral catheter serves as a diagnostic instrument with which one may calibrate the urethra, measure the
amount of residual urine in the bladder and instill opaque
fluid to outline the bladder for a cystogram. The art and science of urethral manipulation and cystoscopic examination
demand a gentle nature, a sympathetic understanding and
manual dexterity. Nowhere in surgery is "tactus eruditis"
more important. A dominant feature of this specialty is the
accuracy of diagnosis afforded by the studies and measurements just outlined. The following quotation from Lord
Kelvin seems especially appropriate for the urologist:

> "I often say that when you can measure what you are
> speaking about and express it in numbers you know
> something about it; but when you cannot measure it,
> when you cannot express it in numbers, your knowledge
> is of a meagre and unsatisfactory kind; it may be the be-
> ginning of knowledge, but you have scarcely in your
> thoughts advanced to the stage of Science, whatever the
> matter may be."

The practice of urology demands the study and management of congenital anomalies, injuries, infections, neoplasms
and metabolic disturbances of the genitourinary system as
well as their complications that may affect the entire organism.
Continued progress in the study of anatomy, embryology and
physiology have aided in the treatment of congenital anomalies. Great strides have been made in the past twenty-five years

in the treatment of infection as a result of the development of the sulfonamides, which was the true beginning of chemotherapy. This was followed shortly by Sir Alexander Fleming's discovery of penicillin, which in its turn was followed by Selman Waksman's development of streptomycin, and by numerous other antibiotics now available. A detailed knowledge of the antibiotics, the indications for their use and the possible complications are especially important to the urologist. All of their particular hazards must be familiar to him and he must at all times be alert to the necessity of changing or discontinuing this type of therapy.

Great improvements have come about during the past decade in the management of renal insufficiency, owing to increased knowledge of biological chemistry and especially of protein and electrolyte metabolism. Improved understanding of renal disease and the pathologic physiology of the circulation has led to better treatment of all of the surgical disorders of the kidney. A detailed understanding of anesthesiology is especially important in this field of surgery since so many elderly patients must undergo operation. The proper choice of an anesthetic agent for the elderly patient with renal failure requires the most careful discrimination and judgment.

Neoplastic disease involving the prostate, bladder, kidneys and testis offers special opportunities for clinical investigation and research. Thanks to the work of Dr. Charles Huggins of the University of Chicago during the last twenty years, the hormonal therapy of cancer beginning with the prostate and progressing to the breasts, thyroid, pituitary and adrenal has been placed on a sound basis. This approach has also led to advances in the over-all study of the chemotherapy of cancer. Since the advent of cortisone and adequate substitution therapy for patients with adrenocortical insufficiency great advances have been made in the surgery of the adrenal glands. The first bilateral total adrenalectomy was successfully carried out by the urologist. His interest in endocrinology is also stimulated by the pheochromocytoma, the parathyroid adenoma, hyperplasia of the parathyroid, hyperplasia of the adrenal cortex and by the functioning tumors of the testis such as the chorionepithelioma, interstitial cell and Leydig cell tumors. An entirely new field of endeavor has developed in the transplantation of tissues, which has for the first time been successfully carried out between identical and non-identical twins by the urologist working with the general surgeon. This has opened up a whole new field of investigation and research both in the laboratory and in the clinic, involving all services of the general hospital and medical school.

The urologist has participated actively in a renaissance of interest in combating environmental sepsis by detailed bacteriologic studies in the cystoscopic room, the operating room, the wards, the clinic and the laboratory. Dr. Carl W. Walter at the Peter Bent Brigham Hospital has led the world in this approach to a fatal problem first emphasized to us by Semmelweis. The urologist has taken a very active part in the investigation of renal hypertension since Goldblatt first discovered that this could be produced in the laboratory by provoking renal ischemia. All patients with accelerated hypertension are studied and treated for renal ischemia by urologists when the latter condition is the cause of the patient's hypertensive vascular disorder. The diagnosis and surgical treatment of renal vascular disease falls naturally into the sphere of the urologic surgeon. At the same time hypertension produced by pheochromocytoma, hyperplasia or tumor of the adrenal cortex is discovered by urologic diagnostic measures and is usually treated by the urologic surgeon. The challenges multiply with progress, which furnishes the opportunities of the present and future. One can only envy him who has the privilege of choosing urology as a career for the next twenty-five years.

Professor William S. Halsted of Johns Hopkins University is the father of the residency training system in surgery in this country. It required three full decades for the residency system to become widely established in the teaching institutions and subsequently in the community hospitals and private clinics. The residency system was established in general surgery and subsequently in the various specialties of surgery. Prior to the establishment of the residency in urologic surgery the training was that of general surgery, which included urology, and those who chose to remain in this field of endeavor limited themselves to that type of practice. Others attached themselves to well-established surgeons who were doing predominantly urologic surgery and served for years as apprentices. Gradually as the residency system has developed the habit of training by an apprenticeship has disappeared. The Board of Urology was one of the earlier surgical specialty boards, being established in 1933; the Board of Surgery followed in 1937. The boards have served the important purpose of certifying men who are fully qualified to practice the various types of surgery that have, of necessity, developed. After the first twenty years the requirements of the different boards have become quite definite and concise. It is significant that Dr. Hugh Hampton Young, appointed as professor of urology at Johns Hopkins University by Professor William S. Halsted, should have developed the earliest full residency in urology in this country. Dr. Young was a pioneer in this specialty and made many important contributions of both scientific and educational value. His was perhaps the first separate department of urology. Squires of Columbia University, Keyes of Cornell, Schmitt of Northwestern, and Kretschmer of the Rush Medical College were all pioneers in the establishment of urologic teaching services.

The present day requirements for certification by the Board of Urology are a year of internship, a year as a resident in surgery and three years in a urologic residency recognized by the Board of Urology, the American Medical Association, and the American College of Surgeons. It is my conviction that those who are planning to have a career in academic surgery are well advised to qualify with the Board of General Surgery as well as that of Urology. A number of young men who have graduated from medical school prior to the age of twenty-four have spent a year or more in internal medicine or in one of the basic sciences in their preparation for urologic surgery.

In all instances of which we are aware this has been a very worthwhile expenditure of time. After finishing the three years of residency in urologic surgery the candidate is required to put in two years in the practice of urology before taking the examinations of the Board. Having completed this qualification for certification by the Board he is eligible to apply for membership in the American Urological Association and the American College of Surgeons. The American Urological Association, which is subdivided into eight geographical sections, is dedicated to education and research as well as to maintaining the highest ideals in the practice of urology.

Urologists in the Regular Army, Navy and Air Force are eligible for membership in the Association. Each of the sections has its own officers and holds meetings each year, with scientific programs, in addition to the single annual meeting of the entire Association. Students, interns and residents are welcome and are encouraged to come to all of the meetings of these organizations. Awards are made annually to residents for outstanding contributions in research in the laboratory and in the clinic. A smaller and older organization than the American Urological Association is the American Association of Genito-Urinary Surgeons, which was initially formed by general surgeons predominantly interested in urology. Members of this organization were in the past half century the actual parents of the specialty of urology and have continued through the years to exert a helpful influence on it. The Board of Urology is composed of representatives of the American Association of Genito-Urinary Surgeons, the American Urological Association and the Urological Section of the American Medical Association. The members of the American Urological Association continue to maintain their interest in the activities of the American College of Surgeons and the American Surgical Association, as is evidenced by continued representation of their members in these organizations. This has a very helpful influence in maintaining the best communications and relations between urology and general surgery. By maintaining such communications it is possible to minimize the development of false barriers between these specialties.

It has been observed that urology continues to be an ever-broadening field of endeavor involving bacteriology, pharmacology, chemotherapy, radiology, endocrinology, vascular disease, urologic diagnosis and genitourinary surgery. The opportunities in this area today are limited only by the individual's imagination.

During the past twenty-seven years at the Peter Bent Brigham Hospital and the Harvard Medical School it has been informative to interview students applying for appointments as surgical house officers. When does one decide to enter internal medicine or surgery as a career? What usually determines this decision? For surgery the decision is usually final after the student's course in fourth-year surgery, though the introduction to surgery in the second and third years may have resulted in an early decision for many.

Choice of a clinical specialty beyond these major fields prior to post-doctorate training is premature and probably not based on sound judgment although the decision for a career in one of the basic sciences may well come in the first two years of medical school. Many students decide that their career will be in internal medicine during the third year though they may change this decision during the fourth year of medical school. The evolutionary process is not a passive one but the role of circumstances in the final choice of a career cannot be denied. The prolonged preparation for an academic career in surgery or one of its specialties carries severe economic implications. The patient moral and sometimes economic support by one's wife through the years often constitutes a determining factor in the choice that is made.

It should be emphasized in closing that in urology as in all other branches of medicine and surgery today the care of the patient is accomplished by a team effort. The day is now gone when the physician or surgeon constitutes the know-all and do-all in his care. One must agree with the concept of modern surgical care as so complex that the welfare and safety of the surgical patient are of necessity best served by competent hospital personnel collaborating under the direction of the atending surgeon.

BIBLIOGRAPHY

Garrison, F. A.: History of Medicine, Philadelphia, Saunders, 1929.

Lewis, B., Ballenger, E. G., Frontz, W. A., and Hamer, H. A.: History of Urology, Baltimore, Williams & Wilkins, 1933.

WILLIAM FEINDEL, M.D.

Professor of Neurosurgery at McGill University

12

Neurosurgery

When Abraham Lincoln was once asked his opinion of a certain book, he replied, "People who like this sort of thing, will find this the sort of thing they like." The comment, though admittedly diffident and laconic, is relevant to the problem of tendering advice to young men and women about to consider a choice among the varied array of specialties open to them in the vast field of modern medicine. The difficult task faced by a physician in describing the nature of his profession to others was discussed some thirty years ago by perhaps the most famous of neurosurgeons, Harvey Cushing, in an address to undergraduates at Dartmouth College.

"In view of the peculiarly intimate nature of their own vocation, practitioners of Medicine, except among their own kind, are traditionally close-mouthed; and since one cannot properly speak of his profession in public without praising it, doctors are inclined to dodge that embarrassing task, preferring to let the amazing developments in Medicine during the past fifty years speak for themselves. What is more, responsibility is added to embarrassment, by the expressed hope that what I may have to say will produce from among you some good physicians and repel some incapable ones. There is, in reality, little to be said, other than that Medicine has become so many-sided that anyone with a good head, a good heart or skillful hands, who is possessed of a spirit of service, who is not afraid of hard work, and who will be satisfied with a modest income, will find ample opportunity for happiness and for the exercise of his talents; and this is doubtless true no less of other vocations."

Those who may be considering neurosurgery as a career may reasonably ask several questions: What is the field of neurosurgery? What is the role of neurosurgery in the general field of medicine? How does one qualify as a neurosurgeon? This brief outline will try to provide some of the answers and to indicate where further information may be found.

THE SCOPE OF NEUROSURGERY

The term "neurosurgery" needs little definition. Its scope includes the surgery of the brain, the spinal cord and the peripheral and autonomic nerves. Necessarily, it involves those structures covering the nervous system, so that surgical lesions of the scalp and skull and lesions of the vertebral column compressing the spinal cord or spinal nerves, such as fracture-dislocation or ruptured intervertebral disks, properly come within the province of the neurosurgeon.

Neurosurgery is an expanding field. A generation ago those devoting their attention entirely to surgery of the nervous system numbered no more than a score. Today, in the United States alone, there are more than a thousand. The training and qualification of neurosurgical specialists is the concern of a separate American Board of Neurological Surgery. There are five national neurosurgical societies. Although their perennially rotating gathering-places may read somewhat like a travelogue, they serve the serious purpose of providing for discussion of training requirements, establishing surgical methods, review of surgical results and of new advances in technics, and, no less important, for the diffusion of professional fellowship.

Another feature of neurosurgery today is its international character, which began after World War I when surgeons from overseas came to study with Harvey Cushing. At present the majority of the senior neurosurgeons of Britain, for example, are disciples of Cushing and there continue to be many examples of this healthy interchange between various countries. Neurosurgeons in various stages of preparation from this continent have always been welcomed at the great teaching clinics of Queen Square, Paris, Stockholm, and many of the other active centers of neurologic study in Europe. On this side of the Atlantic we seem to have an even more active arrangement. At the present time, for example, a Canadian with a background of anatomic research in Holland and neurologic training in Chicago is professor of neurologic surgery at Johns Hopkins. Two young neurosurgeons, Wilder Penfield and William Cone, moved from the United States to Canada some thirty years ago to found with the help of a generous Rockefeller endowment the Montreal Neurological Institute at McGill University. Here, surgeons, neurologists and neurologic scientists from almost every part of the globe continue to come for some part of their training. A continual stream of young neurosurgeons from South America come to do post-graduate work in the United States. The traffic is seldom ever one way. One should note perhaps that a surgeon from Tennessee is now chief of neurosurgery in the Teaching Hospital of Oxford University.

Since the turn of the century neurosurgery has passed through several phases. At first, the surgeon was engaged largely in the struggle to reduce operative mortality. This, in retrospect, seems today like a hand-to-hand struggle, when compared with the remarkable support the surgeon now enjoys from diagnostic methods such as radiology, electroencephalography, excellent anesthesia, well-established operative technics, antibiotics, and specialized nursing care.

With further advances, more daring operative approaches to the brain and spinal cord were developed, and more elective surgery was performed as operative mortality steadily decreased.

Finally, what may be called the investigative phase of neurosurgery became established and surgical treatment began to be applied to disorders where surgical methods had previously been far too hazardous. So active has this development been

in the past decade and so many are the unsolved neurologic problems still awaiting treatment that the future limits
are difficult to define.

Some of the major diseases and disorders that lie within
the scope of neurosurgery will continue to activate further
expansion of this specialty. Head injuries and spinal injuries
are on the increase. Cerebrovascular disease, the third most
common cause of death, and the most common cause of neurologic disability, is in some instances now being successfully
treated by the neurologic and the vascular surgeon. Tumors
of the brain and spinal cord are still problems and will continue to engage the neurosurgeon's attention for years to
come.

Surgical fashions change. Sympathectomy for hypertension
and frontal lobotomy have given way to more successful relief
by medical means. On the other hand, the selective surgical
treatment of focal epilepsy and of involuntary movements
such as parkinsonism has offered relief—often dramatic relief
—where treatment by drugs has failed to give adequate
control.

Finally, in psychiatric disorders, I predict that the neurosurgeon will play an increasing role. As Sherrington has put
it, "The brain and the psyche lie together so to say, on a knife
edge." Already the neurosurgical study and treatment of focal
epilepsy has yielded new insight into disorders of memory,
thought and speech. So long as the neurosurgeon in the course
of therapy is presented the opportunity, unique in the field
of medicine, of observing man's living brain, the onus is on
him, working closely with the neurologist, the psychiatrist
and the neurological scientist, to contribute to our understanding of these diseases of the mind that fill half our hospital beds.

NEUROSURGERY IN HISTORY

Though neurosurgery is correctly regarded as a brain-child
of the intensive specialization of twentieth-century medicine,
the finding of prehistoric skulls with surgical openings in

Peru and France suggests that exposure of the brain may have been one of the earliest forms of surgery.

Head injuries and spinal injuries were also the main concern of the Edwin Smith Papyrus, a remarkable surgical manual on trauma dating back to 3000 B.C. but annotated, edited and rewritten in the seventeenth century B.C. This document is comprised of 48 case reports including examples of skull wounds causing post-traumatic hemiplegia and aphasia. A number of spinal injuries are also described, among which are two cases of quadriplegia following fracture-dislocation of the neck. The reports are methodically arranged under title, examination, diagnosis (often including prognosis) and treatment. The surgeon, advised to palpate and examine a scalp wound in a case of fracture of the skull, feels "something throbbing and fluttering under his fingers like the weak place in an infant's crown before it comes whole." As Dr. Wilder Penfield writes, "When one thinks of the probably septic nature of the surgeon's finger three thousand years before Christ, this digital exploration must send a chill down any neurosurgical spine."

Perhaps the most extraordinary fact about this papyrus is the inclusion, for the first time, of the written symbols for brain, meninges and cerebrospinal fluid. The convolutions of the brain were likened to the corrugated surface of the slag on molten copper. Treatment was primitive and consisted of drawing together scalp wounds by adhesive, and of dressing wounds with fresh meat or with a mixture of grease and honey bound on with linen bandages. In spite of the recognition and handling of head injuries by these early Egyptian surgeons and against popular present-day notions, trepanning of the skull was apparently rarely practiced and there is an almost complete lack of surviving examples.

We must look to the Hippocratic era, about 400 B.C., for the first description of trepanning prescribed in certain types of head injuries. In the second century A.D., Galen must have seen recovery from head injuries since he made the comment, "But I have seen a severely wounded brain healed." This first

note of neurosurgical optimism has been chosen as a motto
to embellish the foyer of at least one present-day neurosurgical clinic!

The Greeks, although they were notable for attributing disease to natural causes, had a meager knowledge of brain anatomy. Aristotle, for example, described the brain as cold, fluid
and bloodless. With the risk of almost certain fatal hemorrhage and infection, opening of the skull in ancient Greek
times must have been a desperate last resort, both for the
patient and the surgeon.

In the seventeenth century, it was Thomas Willis, with his
circle of students and friends, including Richard Lower, who
introduced blood transfusion, John Locke, the physician-phi-
losopher, and Christopher Wren, the architect-astronomer,
who was generally responsible for the first significant foundation stone of modern neurology. In his anatomic studies of
the brain, he classified the cranial nerves, described the vascular heptagon at the base of the brain that still bears his name,
and gave clinical descriptions of myasthenia gravis, hysteria,
convulsions and other neurologic disorders. He deserves the
title of the first neurologist. As Sir Charles Sherrington so
aptly writes, "Willis put the brain and the nervous system on
a modern footing so far as could then be done, combining
medical experience with first-hand anatomical knowledge."

The detailed history of the sporadic efforts at surgical treatment of head and spinal injuries through the eighteenth and
nineteenth centuries has been well described in reviews by
Walker and his students, by Horrax and by Sachs.

THE FIELD OF NEUROSURGERY TODAY

The foundation of scientific neurosurgery dates from the
efforts of Sir Victor Horsley at the turn of this century. Starting his professional career as a surgeon, he studied the localization of function in the nervous system in the experimental
laboratory, developing knowledge of neurophysiology and
operative technic which he applied later toward the first effective surgical treatment of lesions of the brain and spinal cord.

A paper by Horsley in 1890 heralded the beginning of the modern era in neurosurgery. In this paper he listed the various conditions of the brain and spinal cord that he considered at that time as "reasonable and justifiable to attack by surgical interference." This list included depressed fractures, extradural, subdural and intracerebral hematomas, hydrocephalus, post-traumatic headache, brain abscess, meningitis, softening of the brain secondary to vascular disease, tumors, including tuberculoma, gummas and parasitic cysts, focal epilepsy, athetosis, traumatic insanity and congenital defects such as meningocele. Among spinal conditions Horsley considered tumor, certain types of fracture, osteomyelitis, and root section for pain.

This "rather modern-looking list," as Horrax has described it, includes pathologic conditions that still defy adequate neurosurgical treatment and that are still stimulating inquiry into newer surgical technics. This is true of every item in Horsley's list except for those such as tuberculoma and the gummatous lesions, which have been conquered not by neurosurgery but by increasingly effective measures in preventive medicine or specifically therapeutic drugs.

It is of interest to compare the list with neurosurgical practice today. Head and spinal injuries continue to make up an increasingly large proportion of emergency work in any neurosurgical unit. They will undoubtedly continue to do so in this age of massed traffic and manned vehicular missiles. For example, some 75 per cent of the persons involved in car accidents suffer head injury, and brain injury represents one of the commonest causes of death in accidents of this type. In addition there is the prolonged morbidity of individuals surviving serious injury of the nervous system in accidents. If considered from the economic point of view alone they offer potent arguments for a program of prevention. There is no doubt that the neurosurgeon today, almost more than any other specialist, has good reason to encourage prevention of traffic accidents.

Hydrocephalus, described by Celsus in the first century

A.D., still offers a challenge in spite of a number of ingenious technics developed over the past ten years. Tubes with one-way plastic valves direct fluid from the blocked subarachnoid or ventricular spaces into the jugular vein or the right auricle of the heart or into the peritoneal or pleural cavity or from the spinal subarachnoid space into the ureter after removal of a kidney. Nevertheless, even these technics do not always result in a successful outcome nor do we yet know some of the basic causes of hydrocephalus, so that this problem will continue to confront another generation of neurosurgeons.

Although neoplasia is the target for an intensive investigative attack on many fronts, a large part of neurosurgical practice today is still taken up with the diagnosis and surgical removal of tumors of the brain and spinal cord. Horsley, and later Harvey Cushing, relied upon a meticulous neurologic history and examination for localizing the site of craniotomy for tumor removal. Cushing refined the technics of neurosurgery and gradually reduced the operative mortality rate of patients with brain tumors to less than 10 per cent which was much the lowest figure attained up to that time. In the removal of acoustic tumors, still one of the most technically difficult neurosurgical feats, his mortality rate toward the end of his career was less than 5 per cent.

Brain abscess and meningitis, like the other infective lesions of the brain, have greatly decreased in importance with the advent of antibacterial drugs. Historically, the neurosurgical treatment of brain abscess by William McEwen in the latter part of the nineteenth century still stands out as an incredible achievement. Once a common and dreaded sight on the neurosurgical ward, brain abscesses have now become almost rare. The neurosurgeon has also played a significant role in the teamwork resulting in successful treatment of tuberculous meningitis after the method of Cairns and Smith at Oxford. Tuberculomas of the brain are now uncommon except in areas where public health control of tuberculosis has not yet been instituted.

Horsley's list includes the problem of athetosis, which represents but one type of involuntary motor movement offering an exciting new field of neurosurgical treatment today. Curiously enough, it was Horsley, with the brilliant assistance of Clarke, who devised and used in monkeys a stereotaxic grid for precise placement of lesions within preselected deep brain structures. This was the predecessor of modern stereotaxic instruments. Recent advances in this field utilize a high energy beam of sound or radiation which, by eliminating the actual placement of a needle in the brain substance, obviates the danger of serious hemorrhage. These stereotaxic procedures, requiring complex equipment, special anatomic knowledge and painstaking control, and applied especially to the treatment of involuntary movements or intractable pain, are capable of offering relief to a vast number of patients whose symptoms are inadequately relieved by drugs presently available. In this field, too, as in so many other aspects of his work, the neurosurgeon stands in an unusually favorable position to contribute to our understanding of the function of the nervous system.

The problem of pain is perhaps more demanding of the resources of the neurosurgeon than almost any other symptom, calling for his skill as a surgical technician, his knowledge of anatomy, and his understanding, as a doctor, of the emotional problems often related to chronic pain. Here again, many advances have been made since the time of Horsley but many problems also remain to be solved. For example, since the days of Horsley and Cushing selective destructive operations and, more recently, decompressive manipulations, on the ganglion or on the posterior trigeminal root, have been successful in relieving the pain of trigeminal neuralgia. But this empirical success need not lead to complacency, since we are still ignorant of the etiology or pathogenesis of this common and excruciating form of pain. An appropriate reminder for us is provided by the comment of John Fothergill, who first gave a clinical description of trigeminal neuralgia in 1776. "We ought never to cease investigating the most abstruse recesses of nature, nor at the same time forget the narrow limits of our capacity, and the danger of presumption."

As in other medical fields, rapid advances in neurosurgery have often been based on the introduction of new technics in diagnosis or treatment. Beginning in 1920, for instance, one of Cushing's students, Walter Dandy, established the valuable diagnostic procedure of pneumography and ventriculography, by which the subarachnoid and ventricular spaces are visualized on x-ray films. This dramatic innovation gives the surgeon confirmatory and often unique information on the location and size of intracranial lesions. As with other valuable mechanical and laboratory diagnostic technics, it brought with it the ever-present danger of using it as a short-cut to careful history-taking and examination so necessary for the intelligent treatment of neurologic disease.

In 1929, the technic of visualizing the blood vessels of the brain by contrast media injected into the carotid or vertebral arteries followed by rapid serial x-ray films was begun by Egas Moniz and Almeida Lima in Portugal, and very shortly after that by Arthur Elvidge in Montreal and Norman Dott in Edinburgh. This technic, however, came into its own only after another decade had passed when, with the decrease in toxicity of the contrast medium and perfection of percutaneous arterial puncture, the method has become widespread. This method gives valuable anatomic information, particularly for arterial aneurysms, angiomas and vascular tumors of the brain. Indeed, the ease with which angiography may now be performed and the wealth of diagnostic information made available is in striking contrast to the difficulties still to be met in attempting surgical treatment of the vascular lesions so disclosed. Nevertheless, the neurosurgical literature today is composed of a large proportion of reports related to this field of cerebrovascular surgery. The significance of this advance can be better appreciated by considering that in 1921 Harvey Cushing apologized for discussing cerebral aneurysm as "a lesion having such remote surgical bearings."

Artificial hypothermia of the patient to reduce the blood flow and metabolism of the brain and to control otherwise fatal hemorrhage has been an important recent advance. This technic was originally introduced by the cardiac and neurosurgical team in Toronto as an adjunct to the treatment of vascular lesions of the brain. Coupled with the study of brain circulation by extremely rapid serial x-ray film and the recent introduction of radio-active isotopes for measuring the speed and volume of blood flow through the brain, these new methods will allow further exploitation and application of neurosurgical technics for the treatment of vascular lesions of the brain.

Occasionally even a new clinical entity appears on the surgical horizon. This is well exemplified by the problem of ruptured intervertebral disk. Disguised for many years under a variety of terms such as lumbago, sciatica, neuritis, and radiculitis, the pain and motor and sensory paralysis resulting from compression of the lumbar and sacral nerve roots by a protruding intervertebral disk was originally clarified by Mixter and Barr and subsequently by others. As a result surgical treatment of protrusion of lumbar, and to a lesser extent, of cervical disks, has come to make up one of the most common operative procedures in neurosurgery. Myelography, the radiologic visualization of contrast medium in the spinal subarachnoid space, has greatly aided the precise diagnosis of disk lesions and, of course, of spinal lesions in general.

Surgery of the peripheral nerves lies within the field of the orthopedic surgeon, the plastic surgeon and the neurosurgeon. The latter can bring to this problem his interest and knowledge of the physiology and pathology of nervous tissue. Even here, the field is not static. Clinical disturbances of various nerves have been long recognized but are by no means properly understood. Careful clinical study here is still rewarding for the neurosurgeon with a keen interest in peripheral nerve physiology. Two recent examples over the past decade that come to mind are the syndromes of compression of the median nerve in the carpal tunnel and compression of the ulnar nerve in the cubital tunnel.

The surgical treatment of focal epilepsy appears on Horsley's list but suffered for many years from lack of sustained interest. Over the past twenty-five years the concentrated research of Penfield and his group has established this also as a special field of neurosurgical endeavor. Combined with electroencephalographic studies and knowledge of neurophysiology, the surgical treatment of epilepsy is unique in that it has kindled enormously widespread interest today in neurophysiology and has led to the development of technics for surface and depth recording and the experimental study of brain activity. Stimulation of the brain and recording of its electrical activity as a necessary adjunct to surgical treatment of epileptic patients has contributed a wealth of observations on the localization of motor, sensory and speech function in man. The most fascinating of all aspects of the surgical treatment of epilepsy, particularly of a variety associated with neuronal discharge in the temporal lobe, is the bearing that this has on our understanding of memory function and the hallucinatory and psychic phenomena, since in this area the neurosurgeon approaches the vast problem of mental disorder.

NEUROSURGICAL TRAINING

There is perhaps no need to emphasize that adequate training in neurosurgery requires time and sacrifice. This is partially because the neurosurgeon must be a neurologist, neuroanatomist, neuropathologist, and surgical technician with a reasonable knowledge today of electrophysiology, radiology and other special aspects of the nervous system in which he may take a particular interest.

The appropriate program for neurosurgical training has always been a subject for lively discussion. As early as 1907 Sir William Osler, in discussing this, "held that a great deal of skepticism in regard to the value of operation in cases of cerebral tumor was the result of the bicipital condition of neurology." He deprecated operations in these cases at the hands of general surgeons and would have preferred to see neurology a special department, so that "there would not be neurological physicians and surgeons but medico-chirurgical neurologists, properly trained in the anatomical, physiological, clinical and surgical aspects of the subject." This in essence represents the general opinion today.

That brain surgery occupied a good deal of Osler's thoughts and even his dreams is clear from a note that he sent from Naples in 1908 to Harvey Cushing, which read as follows: "Thus far on the trip—glorious place—glorious weather. I wish you were *mit*. I dreamt of you last night—operating on Hughlings Jackson. The great principle you set in cerebral surgery was to create a commotion by which the association paths were restored. You took off the scalp—like a p.m. incision—made a big hole over the cerebellum and put in a Christ Church—whipped cream, wooden instrument and rotated it rapidly. Then put back the bone and sewed him up. You said he would never have a fit again. I said solemnly, 'I am not surprised.' H. J. seemed very comfortable after the operation and bought three oranges from a small Neopolitan who strolled into Queen Square amphitheatre; I have been studying my dreams lately and have come to the conclusion that just one-third of my time is spent in the asylum, or should be!"

Some twenty-five years later, Cushing outlined the requirements of a training program. "It goes without saying that a neurologist should first of all be a good physician; also, that a neurosurgeon would be the better were he primarily well trained as a neurologist. If we grant these premises, the neurosurgeon should first have a general medical training, followed by experience in general surgery before he begins to take up his specialty. How far he will go into neuropathology, neuropsychiatry and experimental neurophysiology while studying to prepare himself in neurology will necessarily depend on his opportunities and ambition to round out his training. If he is to make his own diagnoses—and should he not do so he will miss the chief intellectual interest in his work—he must be a good practical ophthalmologist, otologist and endocrinologist. On top of all this, he must become proficient in the peculiarly detailed ritual of intracranial operations in which comparatively few can ever hope really to excel." It is almost unnecessary to point out that this is a formidable undertaking, requiring perseverance, physical and mental stamina, and a large measure of patience.

From a practical point of view, the program of graduate training for neurosurgical qualifications, as set out by the American Board of Neurological Surgery, requires, beyond the internship, a year of general surgery and four years of residency training which should include at least a year and a half of clinical neurosurgery, six months of basic science and one year of neurology or neurosurgical research. In addition, two years of neurosurgical practice are necessary before the candidate becomes eligible to take the examinations. At the time of the examination he is required to submit a list of all hospital patients for whom he has been the responsible surgeon during these two years. The Board provides a useful outline of the information with which the candidate is expected to be familiar.

A similar course of training is advised by the Royal College of Physicians and Surgeons of Canada leading to written and oral examinations granting Fellowship and qualification as a neurosurgical specialist.

It should be emphasized that advice regarding appropriate training programs should be sought as early as possible from qualified neurosurgeons, so that the requisite portions of the training may be properly planned and approved by the examining bodies.

Needless to say, during the course of his long and strenuous training the candidate will encounter many personal and professional problems, and the practical realization of his hopes may at times appear very distant indeed. It is not unlikely that he will feel occasionally like Alice in *Through the Looking-Glass,* when told by the White Queen, "The rule is, jam tomorrow and jam yesterday but never jam *today.*" He will need to cultivate some of the qualities ascribed to William Harvey—love of truth, reverence, charity, with some tincture of imagination and humor, moral courage, patience and reflectiveness. He will have some consolation in remembering that even Osler, at the time of his final examinations as a medical student, much worried as to the future and partly as to what he should do afterwards, gained solace from Carlyle's admonition, "Our main business is not to see what lies dimly at a distance but to do what lies clearly at hand."

SUGGESTED READINGS

Some of the ablest neurosurgeons have been equally as skillful with the pen as with the scalpel and an excellent idea of the field of neurosurgery can be gained from some of the following references. The delightful essays by Harvey Cushing and the recently published papers of Sir Geoffrey Jefferson will be enjoyed by any reader, medical or non-medical. The textbook of neurosurgery, edited by Dr. Kahn and his associates, gives, I think, the best review of the scope of neurosurgery today. The monograph by Dr. Penfield and Dr. Jasper indicates in a fascinating way the contribution that the neurosurgeon and the neurologic scientist can make to the understanding of the function of the brain. The two charming medical essays by Dr. Penfield will be found thought-provoking. The small volume on memory, learning and language indicates how some of the problems of neurosurgical research relate to the fields of education, automation and psychiatric research. In the final article on the list, Dr. Walker, besides editing the extensive history, takes a fresh look at the field of neurosurgery.

BIBLIOGRAPHY

Cushing, H.: Consecratio Medici and Other Papers, p. 276, Boston, Little, 1940.

Cushing, H.: The Medical Career and Other Papers, p. 302, Boston, Little, 1940.

Fulton, J. F.: Harvey Cushing: A Biography, p. 754, Springfield, Thomas, 1946.

Feindel, W. H. (ed.): Memory, Learning and Language—The Physical Basis of Mind, U. of Toronto Press, 1960.

Horrax, G.: Neurosurgery—An Historical Sketch, p. 135, Springfield, Thomas, 1952.

Jefferson, Sir Geoffrey: Selected Papers, p. 563, London, Pitman, 1960.

Kahn, E. A., Bassett, R. C., Schneider, R. C., and Crosby, E. C.: Correlative Neurosurgery, p. 413, Springfield, Thomas 1955.

Paget, S.: Sir Victor Horsley, A Study of His Life and Work, p. 358, New York, Harcourt, 1920.

Penfield, W.: Neurosurgery yesterday, today and tomorrow, J. Neurosurg. *6*:6-12, 1949.

——: Convocation vistas: a philosophy for doctors, Queen's Quart. *64*:161-169, 1957.

Penfield, W., and Jasper, H.: Epilepsy and the Functional Anatomy of the Human Brain, p. 896, Boston, Little, 1954.

Sachs, E.: The History and Development of Neurological Surgery, p. 158, New York, Hoeber, 1952.

Walker, A. E. (ed.) : A History of Neurological Surgery, p. 583, Baltimore, Williams & Wilkins, 1951.

——: Changing role of neurological surgery in medicine, J.A.M.A. *156*:833-835, 1954.

FRANCIS HEED ADLER, M.D.

Professor of Ophthalmology at the University of Pennsylvania

13

Ophthalmology

Of all the specialties, ophthalmology is nearest to general practice. It embraces general surgery, internal medicine, neurology, dermatology, and even obstetrics. Psychiatry plays a prominent role, since the eye is frequently the organ to which the emotionally disturbed person transfers his complaints, and psychosomatic symptoms are encountered frequently. The ophthalmologist must be a pediatrician and a geriatrist, since he also deals with the special problems of the very young and the very old. Strangely, the specialty with which ophthalmology was closely linked in the early days of its growth in this country, otolaryngology, has the least claim on the ophthalmologist's attention, except for the hardly laudable purpose of increasing his income. The combined practice of eye, ear, nose and throat never had any reason for existence except an economic one, and it is on the way out.

Unlike the general practitioner, the ophthalmologist can become reasonably proficient in his knowledge of each special field, since he confines himself to only those parts of each specialty having to do with one small organ. Many general diseases have characteristic and often pathognomonic ocular changes that enable the ophthalmologist to make a tentative diagnosis. A few examples of these are: the exophthalmos and lid signs of Graves' disease; the Argyll-Robertson pupil in neurosyphilis; the eyeground changes in conditions associated with increased pressure; diabetic retinopathy; and choked disk in brain tumors. The ophthalmologist must know enough general medicine to recognize the eye changes that signify general disorders elsewhere in the body, and yet he need not know all about these entities, and does not have to concern himself with their treatment. Today, new or perhaps only recently recognized diseases are being discovered which involve the eye in characteristic ways. The ophthalmologist must be on his toes to pick up these pathologic changes in the eye and realize their significance. The collagen diseases, disorders of metabolism such as cystinosis, Hurler's disease, Marfan's syndrome and other diseases of connective tissue have diagnostic eye changes. Many of the so-called heredodegenerative diseases of the central nervous system are now thought to have manifestations in the eye. Hence, the ophthalmologist never separates himself from general medicine, and becomes an important member of the diagnostic team.

Unlike the internist, when the ophthalmologist has a patient who requires surgery he does not have to turn him over to a surgeon. Although ophthalmology is often categorized as a surgical specialty, it is far from being so, and there is equal justification for tying it up to internal medicine or neurology. If it is to be linked with surgery, its partner should be neurosurgery and not general surgery, for the eye is an outgrowth of the brain (the optic nerve is a fiber tract of the central nervous system and not a true sensory nerve), and the surgical technics employed are the delicate and refined ones of neurosurgery rather than those of abdominal or orthopedic surgery. A mild tremor is no bar to the general surgeon, but cannot be condoned in an ophthalmic surgeon, who properly has been called the millimeter surgeon, doing most of his manipulations under magnifying glasses. The success or failure of an eye operation generally depends on the manual dexterity of the operator, and the results are always apparent to the patient.

The tragedy of blindness and the enormous importance of sight to the individual makes the practice of ophthalmology exciting and rewarding. To be able to restore sight to an individual who has lost it is more than heart warming. I once had a new young secretary in the office who watched me fit a cataract glass on a patient I had just operated on and who had been blind for a number of years. When the patient shouted with joy, "I can read again!" she burst into tears. All of us share daily in this genuine emotion. If the greatest reward of medicine is to be able to help our fellow men, surely ophthalmology offers us great opportunities.

From this you may conclude that being an ophthalmologist is like being a big frog in a small pond rather than a small frog in a big one. There is a certain feeling of pride that a reasonably complete knowledge of his field is attainable in ophthalmology, and one does not have the discouragement of the general practitioner who, even in late professional life, sees his most interesting cases taken out of his hands and referred to the "specialist."

The beginner in ophthalmology has an economic advantage. At the start his practice is largely refraction and the treatment of minor inflammatory diseases. He does not starve while waiting for his first cataract operation. If he is good with children he soon builds a practice taking care of the refractive errors of childhood, and these patients stay with him through life. He becomes a friend of the family and enjoys the same intimate relation that is the great reward of the general practitioner.

There is no overcrowding in ophthalmology. Outside the smaller cities—those under a hundred thousand population—there is a real scarcity, and refraction is generally done by the optometrist, necessarily without cycloplegia, the more serious ailments being referred by the family doctor to a specialist in some nearby city. This deficiency in the smaller towns is being made up by recent graduates from residences in ophthalmology. With the development of good facilities in the local hospital, better eye care is being afforded the general population outside medical centers. The general public is becoming aware that better eye care is more likely to be secured from a physician who practices ophthalmology alone, and does not combine it with otolaryngology. Once the diploma of the American Board of Ophthalmology has been secured there will be no lack of patients. At the present time there are 5160 diplomates of the American Board of Ophthalmology to take care of 180,000,000 people, so the field is certainly not overcrowded.

Another incentive to become an ophthalmologist is the tremendous growth in the last ten years of interest in the physiology and chemistry of the eye. A most dramatic and exciting series of discoveries in the way the eye functions has developed from the application of modern chemical and electrophysiologic technics. The well-trained young graduate with interest in research and academic medicine is assured a fertile professional field, and the possibility of making important original contributions himself.

Before World War I most of the important work on the chemistry, physiology and experimental pathology of the eye came from Germany. Now the laboratories in this country and in England lead the world and are attracting foreign students by the hundreds. In every large department of ophthalmology research in both the basic study of the eye as a sense organ, and in the cause and treatment of diseases of the eye is being pursued at feverish heat, with no present lack of funds for support. The Section on Neurology and the Blinding Diseases, at the National Institutes of Health, and other foundations are contributing large sums of money for eye research, and for the training of those who show an aptitude for investigative work. Basic scientists are given encouragement to turn to the eye as an organ of research through the development of long term grants-in-aid, and by their employment on a full-time basis by departments and institutes of ophthalmology. Academic ophthalmology is being stimulated by a training-grant program from the Institutes of Health, designed to give an opportunity to those whose talents indicate that they are future professorial timber.

Some of the more important discoveries may be mentioned to illustrate the recent advances that have taken place in the physiology of the eye.

Since Boll discovered rhodopsin, or visual purple, in 1876,

it has been known that some pigment or pigments having selective absorption of light of different wave lengths must be present in every photoreceptor, whether an insect's eye or that of man. Due to the work of many different investigators, but largely to that of George Wald, at Harvard, the pigment rhodopsin has now been not only chemically analyzed, but synthesized in the laboratory, and the cycle through which this pigment is broken down by light and reformed in the dark in the retina largely revealed. The first step in the process of vision has been solved. As a result of the breakdown of rhodopsin by light, energy is released, creating a complex series of changes in electrical potential in the retina, which, when suitably recorded, is known as the electroretinogram. Recent studies by Granit and other workers are succeeding in analyzing this complex electrical change into its component parts, showing where they originate in the retina and what portions are passed on into the optic nerve fibers, whence they are conducted up to the brain as the message of sight. A fairly accurate analysis of what this coded message is and how it changes with changes in the various parameters of the light stimulus has been worked out, so that we now know pretty well the type of message received by the brain. From studies of the electroencephalogram we are making a beginning of what the brain does with this coded message and how it translates this into that form of consciousness that we call sight. These forward steps have been achieved by the application of modern chemical and electrophysiologic technics.

Until recently our knowledge of eye movements has been largely anatomical, plus the information that comes from associating disturbances of motility with the situation of lesions in pathologic specimens. With the modern application of electrophysiology to the muscles themselves we are beginning to acquire new concepts of ocular motility. This will materially aid us in the understanding of ocular muscle palsies, myasthenia gravis and allied conditions, and the problems of strabismus.

The problem of grafting tissues has been applied to the eye

with the dramatic result of successfully transplanting corneas from one human being to another. Permanently clear grafts can now be achieved in the majority of suitable cases, and hundreds of people have had their sight restored by this method after their corneas had been made opaque by disease.

As the result of the development of the gonioscope, a simple instrument by means of which the angle of the anterior chamber of the eye can be visualized, two separate forms of glaucoma, which blinds more people in the United States than any other disease, are now recognized. This has led to the clarification of many puzzling problems, and together with the development of tonography, a method for determining the resistance to outflow of aqueous humor from the chamber angle, has resulted in vastly improved treatment of this dread disease. Electronmicroscopy of the angle is now revealing further facts that may ultimately demonstrate the cause of glaucoma and how to prevent it.

The surgery of the eye has not lagged behind the advances in these other fields. Cataracts are now removed in the lens capsule, avoiding the long period of waiting until the cataract became "ripe." As a result of antibiotics and sutures the dangers of infection, vitreous loss and wound opening are now extremely rare. Detachment of the retina, formerly almost a hopeless condition, is now curable in 75 per cent of the cases operated.

In spite of the disappearance, at least in this country, of blindness due to syphilis, trachoma and tuberculosis, there remain many diseases, particularly those caused by viruses, that offer a challenge to clinical investigation. There are still many forms of blindness that ophthalmology will conquer with the help of inquiring minds.

How does one become trained in ophthalmology? Two ways are open. The best is through a residency training program following a rotating internship in a qualified hospital. The *Journal of the American Medical Association* lists each year those hospitals that have been accredited for residency training in ophthalmology by the Residency Review Committee. This committee carefully inspects and checks regularly on all hospitals offering residencies in ophthalmology to see that certain standards are met. The period of training in these hospitals is at present a minimum of two years, with the vast majority three years, and a few four years. It is likely that within the next year or so the minimum period of training will be set at three years. As with everything else, there are not enough excellent residencies to supply the demand, and an applicant usually applies to several, hoping he will be accepted by his first choice. At present these residencies can be classed into two general types: those given in hospitals run by a medical school, and those in specialized hospitals for either eye, ear, nose and throat diseases, or for ophthalmology alone. More emphasis is being placed now on training in general hospitals affording contacts with the whole field of medicine and surgery, and the few remaining specialized hospitals will probably be forced to affiliate with a general hospital in the not too distant future in order to achieve accreditation.

Following the completion of the residency, a full year must elapse before the candidate can take the examination of the American Board of Ophthalmology. During this year he may practice on his own, or become affiliated with other ophthalmologists, or may elect to spend more time in some form of post-residency training. The Heed Fellowship, for example, enables a man who has completed his residency training to spend six months to a year visiting ophthalmological institutions throughout the country to observe different methods and to engage in research in particular institutions if he so chooses. The National Institutes of Health have established post-residency training grants for the same purpose, and institutes of opthalmology are always on the lookout for promising young men to fill paid full-time or part-time positions in their departments.

The majority of such well-trained men pass the American Board examinations and go into private practice; a few accept full-time salaried positions in departments of ophthalmology, and spend their time in academic pursuits: teaching, research, and departmental administration.

The second approach to ophthalmology is, so to speak, by

the grass-roots method. The individual must get his training in the basic sciences of ophthalmology by either enrolling in the home study courses organized by the Academy of Ophthalmology and Otolaryngology, taking graduate courses in ophthalmology, or both. Numerous graduate courses are offered around the country, running from short one- or two-month courses in certain subjects to a full eight-month course covering the basic sciences and clinical training. These courses are listed every year by the American Medical Association.

Following the completion of such courses of study the individual must wait two years before he can take the American Board examinations. During this period he may practice on his own or become associated as an office or hospital assistant with a diplomate of the American Board of Ophthalmology, who acts as his preceptor.

It is obvious that this latter approach is not as certain of success as that of an accredited residency, since much more depends on the individual's initiative, industry and intelligence, and also on the preceptor and the amount of time he gives to the problem of adequately training the candidate. If he merely uses the candidate as a means of getting his office routine done, and does not take the time and trouble to instruct him, the chances are that the candidate will not be well trained. If, on the other hand, the preceptor is a good teacher, interested in seeing that the preceptee learns as much as possible, the training may be ever better than that afforded by the average residency. The vast majority of failures in the American Board examinations occur in the group of preceptees, but this does not necessarily indict the system, since obviously the majority of the men who take precepteeships are those who were not accepted by the residency training programs. Occasionally one finds the best grades in the examination turned in by a preceptee, showing that it is largely the individual candidate and the individual preceptor that count.

What are the forums of ophthalmology and its scientific journals, where one keeps abreast of new developments and reports of unusual cases? There are four major ophthalmological societies in this country, three of which have a long lineage. The American Ophthalmological Society, founded in 1864, is the second oldest ophthalmological society in the world, antedated only by the Deutsches Ophthalmologisches Gesellschaft. Its membership is limited to approximately two hundred, elected primarily on the basis of their contributions to ophthalmology and the acceptance of a thesis submitted after at least ten years of practice. The Section of Ophthalmology of the American Medical Association was organized in 1878, and is an open forum to all members of the Association and invited guests. The American Academy of Ophthalmology and Otolaryngology, established in 1896, holds not only meetings where scientific papers are read, but also many small conferences, each under the direction of a recognized leader in the field. These are designed as instructional periods and are followed by questions from the group. These stimulating conferences afford a constant opportunity to all for continuing education. The need for a special forum for research in ophthalmology where basic scientists working in ophthalmological fields, as well as ophthalmologists, could present the results of their work, resulted in the formation of the Society for Research in Ophthalmology. Two major periodicals, the *A.M.A. Archives of Ophthalmology* and the *American Journal of Ophthalmology,* have a world-wide circulation.

A word about ophthalmology as a discipline. The ophthalmologist must not only be able to see; he must be able to observe. What he looks at is small, and the pathologic changes may be slight—a speck of dust on the cornea, a slight irregularity in the shape of the pupil, fine vitreous dust, minimal constriction of the small branches of the retinal artery—yet these he must pick up. He must have both good eyes and a well developed power of observation. In addition he should have a retentive visual memory. He need not remember cold facts (they can be found in the books), but he must recall what something looked like a few days or weeks before, and note any changes that have occurred.

It goes almost without saying that he must work hard if he is to do a good job, and to live up fully to his own capabilities. This is no easy way of life. He must be continually aware that his education is never finished, and that studying never stops. A check of reading habits according to specialties at the library of the College of Physicians of Philadelphia showed that the greatest number of books and journals were read by neurologists. Second on the list were ophthalmologists. Although he has few night calls, the successful ophthalmologist after a busy day generally spends the majority of his evenings with his books, papers and records.

FRANCIS L. LEDERER, M.D.

Professor of Otolaryngology at the University of Illinois

14

Otolaryngology

In 1959, the Association of American Medical Colleges sent questionnaires to all students in the June graduating class of that year inquiring about the particular type of practice they intended to follow. Sixty-eight per cent of these questionnaires were returned; less than 2 per cent of those replying were undecided. Sixty-five per cent of the students stated that they intended to enter some form of specialty practice, compared with 26 per cent committed to general practice. Seven and a half per cent hoped to do full-time teaching and research.

For those students who are undecided and for those whose otolaryngologic exposure as undergraduates was meager or indifferent, the final decision is still open. They need the internship and the residency periods in which to decide on a career.

Some students have decided before entering medical school to pursue otolaryngology while others find their way into the field by sheer chance. Family ties to otolaryngologists frequently enter into the selection, for many second generation otolaryngologists have continued in the chosen field of their fathers and some have achieved greater recognition.

A broadened concept of otolaryngology goes beyond the fundamental aspects of diseases of the ear, nose and throat and is a natural extension of its own domain and not an invasion of a province competently covered by others.

The subdivisions of this field—otology, laryngology, rhinology, broncho-esophagology and maxillo-facial surgery have reflected the advances in all areas of general medicine and surgery—biochemistry, microbiology, neurology, oncology, ophthalmology, pathology, diagnostic and therapeutic radiology and thoracic and cardiovascular surgery.

It is not generally appreciated that otolaryngology has a rich historical heritage, although one should bear in mind that specialization, as we recognize it today, is of relatively recent origin. Through the ages, however, concern has been expressed that it could lead to no good if a physician restricted himself to one field. Since similar pronouncements have been voiced even to the present day, it is of interest to note them in passing, in the light of the tremendous modern progress in the specialty. In the fifth century before Christ, Herodotus, referring to the Egyptian physicians of that era, stated "The art of medicine is thus divided among them: medicine is practiced among them on a plan of separation; each physician treats a single disease and no more; thus the country swarms with medical practitioners, some undertaking to cure diseases of the eye, others of the head, others again of the teeth, and some, those which are not local." Apparently Montaigne did not share or approve these views of Herodotus for he said "The Egyptians were right in neglecting the general calling of the physician and of dividing the profession; for each illness, for each part of the body, there was an attendant, and therefore each part was more skillfully and less blindly treated, because they studied each one specially."

It is a fact that specialization at various times has been attacked, condemned, and extolled, and startling controversies have dotted the literature of time even to this very day. However, as Owen Wangensteen told the American College of Surgeons in 1946 on the subject of "The Surgeon and His Trust," "There are still a few surgeons who affect to believe that they can take all of surgery for their province. They know as well as anyone that their performance in such a wide category of operative procedure is substandard in some of these areas, when judged in the critical light of what constitutes good practice. Let us be thankful that the day of the all around surgical specialist is done! Surgery is not advanced by that type of activity and no matter how talented the surgeon, he cannot do equally good work in all of these provinces."

The modern "Do-it-yourself" approach to the education of the undergraduate has its limitations. Armed, as he is, with an array of instruments, including an otoscope, a tuning fork, a head mirror and a few mechanical aids that make up an impressive kit, he still needs to be taught their use by those who themselves are skilled in their handling and in the interpretation of the findings. The myth that one man can do all things to all people and do them satisfactorily, is reminiscent of the Marine Corps methodology of creating a fearless, invincible warrior by instilling the belief that a marine can do anything he attempts. The prospective generalist in medicine, while not equipped with such instruments for committing mayhem as an automatic rifle or machine gun, might just as well be, for the results of unskilled application of even diagnostic instruments can result in adverse emotional and physical experiences for the patient. Observing senior medical students, two weeks before convocation, still unable to visualize an oropharynx raises questions regarding the future of the physician and the well-being of the patient. Had the students been better indoctrinated by enthusiastic teachers, it is probable that more of these undergraduates would have elected to enter otolaryngology.

Otolaryngology affords excellent opportunities for the undergraduate student to become acquainted with technics that enable him to examine body recesses and spaces frequently overlooked because of their apparent inaccessibility. The opportunity to acquire such skills and experience is in direct proportion to exposure to the supervision of trained otolaryngologists. Inasmuch as the head and neck contain all of the special senses, knowledge of the structures involved and their functions is paramount. The trend we have advocated has been toward systematizing the knowledge in the field of otolaryngology on the basis of commonly encountered symptoms and signs and to correlate and integrate the basic knowledge of morphology and function. This can be accomplished by presenting the underlying pathologic physiology along with the particular symptoms. Attention is focused on the organ systems but not to the exclusion of the patient as a person and in reference to his environment.

The integration of otolaryngologic information into other medical and surgical disciplines is the purpose of those who try to serve the whole community. It has been estimated that from 30 to 45 per cent of general practice relates to the various disciplines encompassed by otolaryngology. It is of importance that this is recognized by the undergraduate because a general internship may not provide the necessary additional experience. For example the differential diagnosis of swellings about the face and neck are made exactly when the interior of the nose, nasal accessory sinuses, nasopharynx and larynx are routinely inspected by the skilled examiner. The clinical significance of hoarseness becomes a preoperative surgical "must." Impaired motility of a true vocal cord in one case may indicate a tumor of the thyroid gland; its recognition in another may anticipate and discourage legal action precipitated by alleged injury of the recurrent laryngeal nerve. Membranes and ulcerations lend themselves to clearer interpretation when visualized under the direct and indirect means available to the trained eye, not only for inspection but also for biopsy. The same may be said of the tracheobronchial tree and the esophagus, which come in for a share of the otolaryngologist's experience in the field of bronchoesophagology. Peroral endoscopy has outgrown its limited sphere of usefulness in removal of foreign bodies from the air and food passages. Indications for this procedure include various lesions of the tracheobronchial tree and esophagus. The maintenance of the airway is of prime importance in many medical and surgical states. Knowledge of the technic of intubation and tracheotomy are of paramount importance in emergency management. Control of hemorrhage from the nose and throat provokes harrowing experiences on the part of the patient and frustration on the part of the unskilled and untrained physician.

The ear and temporal bone come in for considerable attention as a source of fever, as a disordered mechanism of equilibration or of hearing or both. Functional examination of the vestibular and cochlear systems may yield information on processes that might otherwise be treated as gastrointestinal disorders; or, as in the case of children, hearing loss is mistaken for mental retardation. Otologic microsurgical procedures are now employed to restore useful auditory function in persons with certain types of hearing loss. Not only is recognition of communication disorders stressed through the teaching of audiology but the basic rehabilitative approach affords a pattern fundamental to other sensory types of loss. Diagnosis of the defect is established and the social, educational, psychological, economic and vocational implications of hearing loss are evaluated by a co-ordinated effort of medical and nonmedical workers. The otolaryngologist, in consequence of ever-increasing demands, has been a leader in the development of programs for the hard of hearing and the deaf in military and civilian groups throughout the country.

Since surgery is not only just a technic but is also a method of thinking, and inasmuch as surgery is best entrusted to those who have an intimate knowledge of function and structure, rhinologic and otologic plastic and reconstructive surgical procedures find a natural place in this specialty. Tumors of the head and neck are detected sooner today because of the skill of the otolaryngologically oriented physician. Moreover, with his more adequate knowledge of structure and function, he has a decided advantage over those who have not been so indoctrinated. Tumors of the nose and sinuses, salivary glands, neck, pharynx, larynx and ears are diagnostic and surgical challenges in the domain of the otolaryngologist who possesses the training and experience essential for rational management. In this regard, one is reminded of statements of

Sir Heneage Ogilvie: "The training of a surgeon, at any rate
of one who is to be more than a journeyman operator, begins
after he has taken a higher surgical degree. Knowledge must
be increased, wisdom must be acquired, originality must be
developed, the ability to speak and write must be learnt by
constant practice, and operative experience and technical
skill must be gained by apprenticeship. These things cannot
be found in books. They cannot be self-taught by the isolated
surgeon undertaking responsibility without supervision. They
can be learnt only by the methods by which every art is
learnt, the personal contact of disciple and teacher."

Through the years since Horace Green established himself as the first throat specialist and in 1846 published his
Treatise on Diseases of the Air Passages, otolaryngology
has demonstrated dynamic growth. It has never remained
static but has been able to meet the fresh challenges that have
arisen. It has been the beneficiary of scientific and technological advances, remaining ever alert to the changing medical horizons. The second oldest of the examining boards,
established in 1924, the American Board of Otolaryngology
has led to higher standards of practice of the specialty. It
has demanded basic and clinical training of a superior type
offered only by the better teaching institutions and hospitals
in North America. The aspiring young physician who seeks to
qualify himself in otolaryngology should aim high in his
training. This will be reflected immediately when he becomes
a practitioner dependent on his own resources and when he is
being considered for hospital staff positions and for teaching
appointments.

Finally, it should be emphasized that otolaryngology, more
than some of the other specialties, comprises a field that
ideally lends itself to laboratory and clinical research and to
creative therapeutics. It is true that the pioneers of old had
opportunities and took advantage of them as best they could.
However, these pioneers did not live in the antibiotic era
or in the electronic or space age. Developments of the past
three decades have opened up new avenues and have revealed

new areas to explore. The problems require deeper thinking and increased skill for solution. The young graduates of today should be able to meet these challenges. As a matter of fact, he who dedicates himself to medicine must be able to cope with the problems entailed in such a career. Medicine must have men of good mental stamina!

The broadened scope of otolaryngology, the modern trends, the newly created problems, the opportunities for investigation and study and further development of the specialty—all these opportunities lie before those who contemplate otolaryngology as a career.

BIBLIOGRAPHY

Lederer, F. L.: Objectives in undergraduate teaching, Tr. Am. Acad. Ophth. & Otol. *58*:779-786, 1954.

——: That Part of Your Education for Which You Received No Formal Training. Address, Commencement exercises of the University of Tennessee to graduates in medicine, pharmacy, dentistry, nursing biological sciences, and the graduate school, The Medical Units Division, Memphis, Sep. 27, 1954.

——: Otolaryngological Heritage, Presented before the American Rhinologic Society, Chicago, Oct. 19, 1957.

——: Introduction to Symposium, Are We Good Teachers?, Tr. Am. Acad. Ophth. & Otol. *63*:778-811, 1959.

——: The development of otorhinolaryngology and bronchoesophagology, J. Internat. Coll. Surgeons *33*:83-97; *33*:229-247, 1960.

Lederer, F. L., and Schoolman, J. G.: Postgraduate training in otolaryngology, Arch. Otolaryng. *50*:59-80, 1949.

FRED JENNER HODGES, M.D.

Professor of Radiology at the University of Michigan

15

Radiology

Since the basic, all-pervading motivation of human endeavor is the desire for happiness, it is tremendously important for young people to demand that the lifework of their choice shall promise to them the measure of happiness that they seek. False starts can be extremely costly and are to be avoided because the span of a productive career, from high school graduation to eligibility for social security, is brief, can never be repeated and, in medicine, must include required years of higher education and specialized training.

Those who have been attracted to the medical profession have chosen a field of endeavor within which large numbers of disciples with widely varying interests and talents are needed and can be assimilated. For devoted service rich rewards are assured, both material and in terms of happiness and personal gratification. The practice of medicine takes many forms, including a considerable number of sharply differing fields of specialization, which offer virtually limitless outlets for individual tastes and capabilities. Medical practice may be active or sedentary, practical or theoretical; it may be directly or only remotely related to individual problems of health. It remains for each to select the particular path he wishes to follow throughout his medical career. The prospect of practicing medicine within the field of radiology should appeal to a select number when they have examined the scope, the particular interests and the future prospects of this specialty.

The medical importance of radiation dates from the discovery of x-rays by W. K. Roentgen, professor of physics at the University of Würtzburg, in November, 1895. It was he who first showed that bones within the hand could be photographed with the new invisible penetrating rays. Knowledge concerning the effects of radiations upon living tissues came later and led to their adaptation to therapeutic use. Within the limitations of the primitive apparatus available at the outset, great strides were made during the first decade toward the broad utilization of the newly found method of visualizing hidden anatomic structures.

At the beginning of World War I the use of x-rays in the practice of medicine was sufficiently well established and widespread in this country to warrant the creation of an army school of roentgenology for the training of officers in what was emerging as a new specialty. Physicians who had pioneered in the field and had begun to transmit their knowledge and skills to others were brought together by the Army as the first faculty of the newly organized x-ray school at Camp Greenleaf in Chattanooga, Tennessee. From this beginning the ranks of physicians devoted to medical radiology have been renewed and expanded by ever more thoroughly prepared radiologists turned out by numerous training centers in medical schools and hospitals throughout the country. In 1934 the American Board of Radiology was established under the guidance of many of the very men who had served in the wartime Army school as teachers. As of 1960 more than 6000 candidates have been granted certification by the board in some phase of radiology on the basis of its searching examinations for the determination of fitness.

From the earliest days of the application of radiations to the purposes of medical diagnosis and treatment, the growth and development of the specialty has been vigorous and constantly accelerating in character. Greatly improved apparatus and photographic and opaque materials especially designed for radiologic purposes have broadened the usefulness of radiologic technics, and human ingenuity has conceived new uses, which in turn have stimulated important innovations in equipment design and versatility.

Whenever it has seemed that radiology has reached the upper limits of its usefulness to medicine, some new point of departure has developed as the result of newly available x-ray apparatus, newly perfected surgical procedures, or new observations concerning reliable x-ray signs of disease. Thus a further spiral of increased interest and expansion has been initiated. There is no indication that growth and expansion of the specialty is slackening. Whereas it has always been the case that physicians in various subdivisions of medical practice have to some extent relied upon their own knowledge and ability in utilizing radiation technics within their particular fields, rather than that of trained radiologists, this occasional crossing of specialty borderlines involves relatively few individuals and accents the need for radiologists with highly particularized skills.

There are four major spheres of interest within the broad scope of radiology: diagnostic radiology, therapeutic radiology, radiation physics and radiobiology. Superlative ability in all four divisions is not to be found or to be expected in any one person. Whereas throughout Europe diagnosis and therapy are so completely disassociated as to represent entirely separate and even unrelated specialties, in the United States the majority of radiologists combine these two interests in their practices. As radiologic practice in hospitals, in private clinics and in private offices grows in volume, the tendency for radiologists to restrict their activities to narrower limits of interest becomes apparent. It is not only possible but probable that in this country diagnostic radiology and radiation therapy will become separate specialties before many more years have passed. Still further compartmentalization of particular interests, abilities and experience is to be expected within each of these broad fields.

Many radiologists of national prominence in years past have been known as particular authorities in chest, gastrointestinal, urological or skeletal diagnosis even though their work was not strictly confined to one of these fields. Today several distinct subspecialties are well recognized among diagnostic radiologists because of the great mass of clinical and technical knowledge required if these fields are to be efficiently cultivated. Neuroradiology, pediatric radiology and cardiovascular radiology all represent subdivisions of the diagnostic branch to which one must devote virtually undivided attention and energy if maximum performance is to be expected. The diagnostic use of the radioactive isotopes constitutes another rapidly growing specialized clinical activity in which the American Board of Radiology offers certification on the basis of examinations.

As yet, with but few exceptions, radiation therapists engage in all aspects of this type of practice, devoting themselves exclusively to the treatment rather than the diagnosis of disease. This branch of radiology calls for an entirely different background of clinical knowledge and experience than that which is needed in the various diagnostic divisions, and the daily activities are correspondingly different. Radiation therapy suffers in excellence of quality when it is of necessity practiced in conjunction with diagnosis. With the advent of new sources of useful radiation possessed of sharply differing qualities it may well be that subspecialties in radiation therapy will become logical and desirable.

The continuing development of new apparatus, the ever-present need for accurate dosage determination and efficient protection of people against undesirable exposure provide a broad and interesting field of endeavor for physicists within the framework of medical radiology. People with this type of training and interest are indispensable to the sound and efficient conduct of radiologic practice.

Radiobiology can, and often does, flourish entirely apart from the activities of clinical radiology. As in the case of radiation therapy, outstanding performance demands complete devotion to the technics and the philosophy involved. However, despite their wide differences of interest and activity diagnosis, therapy and physics are properly concerned with basic matters of biologic behavior in response to radiation. An ever-present reminder of potential biologic damage is strengthened by awareness of the results and the implications of current radiobiologic experimentation.

Available openings in the various walks of medical radiology continue to increase at a rate that exceeds the annual output of the training centers. This has been true for the past quarter of a century, and there is no indication that the saturation point has been reached or soon will be. The reasons for this state of affairs seem to be quite apparent. One of the requirements for the approval of a general hospital for internship training is that the full-time services of a radiologist shall be available. Since there are more than 5000 general hospitals in the country, a very sizable pool of radiologists is required to meet their needs alone.

Private practitioners of radiology need professional assistants and associates, and medical schools are constantly in need of radiologists to fill new posts and to replace losses. Occupational medicine provides a growing number of new opportunities, which applies also to health centers developed by industry and labor and by governmental and industrial research institutes. Many excellent and attractive openings have long been available and unfilled in relatively small communities where social and professional life could be most pleasant and rewarding for an able radiologist.

Whereas there is nothing to prevent any physician from providing himself with the necessary apparatus and declaring himself to be a radiologist, his lack of basic training and experience would shortly place serious limitations upon his usefulness and future prospects. It is the effectiveness of preparation rather than the documentary evidence of Board certification that is of primary importance to a radiologist and to the patients he serves.

The basic training requirements of the American Board of Radiology are the result of long experience. By and large, there has been a well-defined correlation between inadequate basic training and failure to pass the Board's examinations.

Currently, candidates for certification must have had three years of postgraduate training in a Board-approved center following internship and must have had one additional year in continuation of their training or in practice. Military service during or after the three basic years is acceptable in fulfillment of the fourth year, provided that the candidate was engaged in approved radiologic activities in a military installation.

Six months of specialized training in pathology is included in the basic period. Experience with many candidates for radiologic training has shown that exposure to any medical discipline over and beyond twelve months of internship can be highly valuable as a broadening and maturing influence. Advanced preliminary preparation in physics, chemistry, or mathematics or a residency year in medicine, surgery, or obstetrics provides great advantages to trainees who later gravitate into subspecialties of radiology where background material in those fields is pertinent. In addition to pathology, some time spent in physiology, anatomy or biochemistry beyond undergraduate requirements can represent a very valuable asset to a radiologist. Previous experience in general practice seems to have lesser value.

Postgraduate radiologic training as prescribed by the Board must provide one year of radiation therapy, including instruction in radiation physics. If certification in isotopic medicine is desired by the candidate, minimum training requirements in this field are stipulated. In general, trainees should be thoroughly instructed in the operation of x-ray apparatus and the handling of radium and radioactive isotopes, including the computation and the measurement of doses delivered. They must be thoroughly indoctrinated in the principles and the practice of radiation protection.

Beginning with instruction by example and followed by closely supervised participation, candidates are introduced to fluoroscopic technics and to the interpretation of films. Gradually, as experience and confidence are attained, greater and greater freedom of action is permitted and encouraged until they can take over a designated part of the departmental load. Graduated responsibilities in radiation therapy range from helping with the setting up of patients and apparatus to checking filtration and dosage, history-taking, patient examination, reporting of treatment administered, treatment planning, radium packaging and placement, and finally first assistantship to the therapist in all daily activities, including the participation in interdepartmental conferences.

Throughout the entire training period the candidate is required to participate in the maintenance of the indexed film library, to study its entire contents and to prepare discussions on some approved subjects for presentation at departmental staff meetings. He is also required to participate in the preparations for interdepartmental clinical conferences and to assist with the student teaching program. Initially, able and well-prepared students who enter upon a program of this sort learn rapidly and become able and useful radiologists before the end of the basic period.

The minimum of five years which must intervene between graduation from medical school and eligibility for Board examination represents a low income period that appears ominously rugged to would-be trainees, especially to those who already have families. Actually, the situation is not an impossible one, for training stipends at most teaching centers come close to providing stark necessities during internship and residency years, and *locum tenens* jobs during parts of vacations pay very well. If the trainee elects to spend the required fourth year in practice, opportunities are numerous, and even before certification he will earn enough to help offset indebtedness incurred earlier. Above all else, the fledgling radiologist should remind himself that the lean years of training lead certainly and surely to a very comfortable income upon the completion of the required period of preparation; an income that will be payable beginning thirty days after training is completed without the necessity of capital investment. Many opportunities in partnership with older associates provide for regularly increasing participation in the net returns from the practice from which the purchase of a share of the partnership is financed over a period of three to five years. In view of the rapid development of financial independence, once preparation has been achieved the privations of a few years should not be too burdensome.

Every young radiologist must decide for himself to what extent he wishes to engage in office or in hospital practice, whether he desires complete independence or the association of other radiologists, or whether perhaps he looks to an academic career. Fortunately, a wide variety of arrangements is available under which he may find the one best suited to his desires and ambitions. He will do well to begin to ponder such matters before the end of his training period. Numerous changes of location and practice arrangements are undesirable unless the advantages are very great, because they interfere with the establishment of a sound reputation. It is wise to consider one's first move into practice with great care and to place long-range advantages well above the matter of initial income level. It is possible to be utterly miserable with a large income if the professional climate is intolerable. One must be able to respect and admire his partner or associates. No contract, however cleverly drawn, is valuable if either party feels it to be unfair. Having accepted appointment as radiologist to a hospital, one should accord that institution full respect and allegiance until the arrangement is discontinued.

A career in medical radiology that is based on sound training and mature planning at the outset can be thoroughly enjoyable and rewarding from beginning to end. Radiology touches intimately almost every other activity in clinical medical practice, providing an opportunity for daily contact with current practices and developments throughout the profession. Within this specialty one can have as much or as little direct contact with patients as he chooses. It is possible to budget time to a considerably greater degree than in many specialties. Hospital practice brings the radiologist into contact with virtually every interesting medical situation within the institution and involves him with many problems of patient care that are never encountered in office practice. If his activities are restricted to a single institution, the time and the energy saved by the elimination of much daily travel that many physicians must accept greatly increases the productivity of the radiologist.

The national radiologic societies include in their activities well-conducted instruction courses and excellent scientific exhibits and have presented at their meetings carefully selected papers dealing with every phase of radiologic interest. Regular attendance at one or more of these annual gatherings and reading the excellent journals that the societies publish provides radiologists with the means of maintaining close touch with new developments even though they may practice in communities remote from teaching centers.

As presently practiced, radiology is interesting, variegated and exciting. The prospect of things to come in the way of phenomenally ingenious technical developments is nothing short of thrilling. It is thoroughly possible that fluoroscopy conducted in dark rooms will be entirely replaced with devices for electronic image amplification that will be far more efficient than anything we have yet seen. The incorporation of television technics promises one day to eliminate the need for costly film consumption, processing and filing by the utilization of video tape recording. These and other technical innovations will in every instance be accompanied by reduction in the radiation exposure to which patients and radiologists are presently subjected. The enormous importance of the contributions of radiology to the diagnosis and the treatment of disease ensures that active and inventive refinement of instruments and adaptations will continue at ever-increasing tempo, as it has throughout the 65 years since Roentgen's discovery.

JAMES E. ECKENHOFF, M.D.

Professor of Anesthesiology at the University of Pennsylvania and Editor of the Journal Anesthesiology

16

Anesthesiology

Although the first public administration of an anesthetic for the performance of a surgical operation occurred nearly 115 years ago, only recently has any large number of physicians become sufficiently identified with anesthesia to be known as specialists. For nearly a century in America, the administration of an anesthetic was considered primarily a technical problem to be managed by nurses, dentists, or relatively untrained physicians. One does not have to seek far to explain why so few physicians became specialists in anesthesia. The nineteenth century was the era of anatomy and pathology. There was relatively little interest in physiology and pharmacology. Those giving anesthetics were too involved in the practical aspects of giving a drug to worry about explanations of drug action or to explore the limitations of the drug. Neither pulse nor blood pressure was monitored or recorded routinely. Only reasonably healthy individuals were thought fit for operation, and generally only simple operations were performed. There was little to attract a physician to a career in anesthesia. An additional deterrent to specialization in anesthesia has been described by Wigodsky: "His (the surgeon's) dominance did little to allow development of anesthesiology, and it is questionable how much encouragement he offered. Apparently, he was content so long as his patient did not yell with pain, did not die from the anesthetic and

did not have a too difficult postoperative course. He expected
the anesthetist to precede him to the operating room, have
the patient asleep when he approached, and leave the rest to
the Lord and himself."

During World War I the situation began to change. Surgical procedures became more complex, and greater demands
were made on the anesthetist. Inquiring minds began to seek
answers to puzzling questions. New and potent anesthetics became available. The equipment for administering anesthetics
improved. Interest in physiology and pharmacology increased.
More and more physicians became identified as anesthetists.
Societies were formed for the discussion of common problems
in anesthesia. By World War II, two journals devoted exclusively to anesthesiology were being published in the United
States, an examining board for certifying specialists in the
field had been established, and there were nearly 2000 anesthesiologists on the membership roles of the American Society
of Anesthetists. The membership of the American Society of
Anesthesiologists now numbers nearly 7000.

The day when a single figure could dominate all aspects
of a surgical patient's care drew to a close. Teams were formed
composed of more than one surgeon, physicians representing
other specialties, and nurses. The development of new anesthetic agents, adjuvants, and technics changed anesthesia into
virtually a new discipline that was beyond the training or
interest of most surgeons. Nor did time permit surgical residency programs to educate surgeons sufficiently in anesthesiology to enable them to supervise adequately the administration of an anesthetic. Therefore, most surgeons welcomed
physician anesthetists as part of the surgical team.

It soon became apparent that an anesthesiologist had much
more to offer than skill in the deliberate narcotization of
patients for surgical operations. He was perforce knowledgeable in the management of unconsciousness, regardless of its
cause. Therefore, his services were requested for patients
comatose from narcotic or barbiturate overdose, cerebral
trauma or vascular accident, hypoxic brain damage, or meta-

bolic derangements such as diabetic coma and uremia. In addition, he became a specialist in resuscitation, both cardiac and respiratory. Indeed, investigations by anesthesiologists led to changing the manual forms of artificial respiration taught to laymen to the simpler, more efficient mouth-to-mouth method of resuscitation.

Anesthesiologists naturally had to study respiration because many anesthetic agents enter and leave the body by way of the lungs and because reasonably normal pulmonary function is essential for the maintenance of the patient's well-being during anesthesia and operation. Some of them became in time authorities on pulmonary physiology, and their advice was sought in consultation for both medical and surgical patients with respiratory problems. Such problems included adequacy of pulmonary exchange, thinning and removal of respiratory tract secretions, decrease in airway dead space, and inhalational therapy in general.

It had long been known that pain relief for surgical operations could be provided by means other than the inhalation of gaseous or volatile anesthetics. Regional anesthesia, without the loss of consciousness, could be provided by the injection of local anesthetics either in the subarachnoid or the epidural space, into nerve trunks, or infiltrated into areas through which incisions were to be made. It became obvious that an anesthesiologist's skill with the needle need not be confined to patients for operation. Various nonsurgical maladies were amenable to nerve block, and regional nerve blocks could be of value in predicting what relief could be expected from operation. Some anesthesiologists established pain clinics, evaluated local anesthetics and published detailed observations on pain and its relief. In the evaluation of other modes of providing relief of pain and discomfort, anesthesiologists have played leading roles. Some have been concerned with major investigations of the actions of narcotics, analgesics, sedatives and tranquilizers.

The introduction of muscular relaxant drugs into clinical medicine revolutionized the practice of anesthesiology. Where once profound general anesthesia or subarachnoid block had been the only ways to provide muscular relaxation, the relaxant drugs provided the means of allowing complete relaxation with minimal anesthesia. The use of curare and allied substances stimulated extensive investigation into the physiology and the pharmacology of the nerve-muscle junction. Much of this fundamental work was carried out by anesthesiologists. Certain diseases such as myasthenia gravis influence the response to muscular relaxants. This not only presents a problem in managing surgical patients with this syndrome but anesthesiologists frequently assist in the diagnosis of myasthenia. Several anesthesiologists have figured prominently in the care of patients with this malady. Even in the myospastic diseases, anesthesiologists can assist in diagnosis and care. In tetanus, anesthetists may assume the major burden of patient care.

Finally, considerable interest has been aroused by the use of hypnosis as a form of pain relief for chronic painful states, or during conditions where only analgesia is required (as in changing burn dressings), and more recently as a method of pain relief during major surgery. A few anesthesiologists are experienced hypnotists, and more are exploring the usefulness of the technic. The field is relatively uncharted, but there may be a wide practical application for hypnosis within the confines of anesthesiology.

From the foregoing, it should be apparent that the interests of anesthesiologists have, in many instances, carried them far afield from the operating room. A few decades ago they were technicians, administering one of several anesthetics to patients whom they had never seen before and probably would not see again, for operations that were for the most part technically simple. They were seldom found outside the operating room.

Today the picture has changed. The anesthesiologist participates in patient care before and after operation as well as during the procedure itself. He is a respiratory physiologist and a clinical pharmacologist. He makes significant contributions to the care of patients suffering from many diseases and complications of diseases. He is interested in fields unrelated to anesthesia and operation. His scope of activity is limited only by his own inquisitiveness and energy.

Anesthesiology is a young specialty. Its confines are not yet clearly drawn. It is in the enviable position of being unable to fill the positions that are available. Therefore, it follows that attractive situations are open in all parts of the country. In no other area of medicine does a physician have such intimate contact with so many other specialties as in anesthesiology. The list includes all the surgical specialties, and also obstetrics, pediatrics, all fields of internal medicine, and radiology. For this reason the anesthetist is likely to stay abreast of the advances being made in many sections of medicine. He is associated with some of the dramatic advances in surgery and the surgical specialties. He is probably in closer contact with the basic sciences than is any other clinician.

Most anesthesiologists confine their efforts to one hospital. This affords opportunity for efficient use of time and permits close patient supervision through constant attendance. Because of this ready availability, anesthesiologists have been designated "Chief of Operating Room" in many institutions, a title that carries with it disadvantages as well as advantages. Most anesthesiologists practice in some form of group practice or partnership which allows rotation of call schedules and assures the members of the group freedom during hours not on duty.

Finally, anesthesiology affords a unique opportunity to make use of mechanical and electronic devices in monitoring patients' vital functions. It is becoming common for anesthetists to monitor the electrocardiogram, the electroencephalogram, blood pressure, heart rate, auscultatory heart sounds, oxygen hemoglobin content, electromyogram, oxygen and carbon dioxide tensions, respiratory gas exchange and anesthetic gas tensions. In no other area outside the physiology laboratory is such monitoring likely.

Each anesthesia is in essence a pharmacologic experiment.

No two patients respond to anesthetics alike. Nowhere else are patients given drugs in such doses as to bring them close to death, yet with such control that recovery with slight deviation from the norm is almost a certainty. There is great satisfaction in anesthetizing desperately ill patients and having them do well. It is under such circumstances that the professional competence of the anesthesiologist, as compared with the technician, becomes so evident.

The clinical practice of anesthesiology has been considered by some to be too routine and to lack intellectual challenge. Perhaps much of clinical anesthesia is routine, but is this not also true of all clinical medicine? In any practice a high percentage of a physician's time is spent on routine problems. How much of a pediatrician's day is spent in examining normal healthy infants and children, in giving prophylactic injections, or in treating minor upper respiratory infections? So it is with anesthesiology. Most patients will be healthy, most will have elective or reasonably straightforward operations, and most will recover from both anesthesia and operation without incident.

The anesthesiologist must have certain personality traits for successful practice. He must not seek to dominate those with whom he works. He must understand that the patients' care is primarily the responsibility of the surgeon: when to operate, the procedure to be undertaken, and in general the course of treatment must be decided by the surgeon. This is not to say that the anesthesiologist has no obligations, for, in the eyes of the law, the physician anesthetist is responsible for all aspects of the administration of the anesthetic. Successful operations today are best performed by teams of physicians. All members of the team must work in harmony and with mutual respect for each other's abilities and opinions, for the benefit of the patient. There is little place for the prima donna. Physicians with such traits should seek a career elsewhere. However, an anesthetist must be quick thinking, be able to reason under pressure and to act decisively. Hypoxia, hypotension and cardiac arrest do not respond to the hesitant and unsure. The management of anesthetic emergencies is not for the individual who functions slowly.

Prolonged patient contact appeals to some physicians and not to others. Anesthesia is a specialty principally associated with acute diseases, and although patients may return for other reasons, repeated visits over the years are unlikely. The exception would be in the case of the anesthetist who engages in the treatment of painful disorders. As a rule, however, the anesthetist does not build up a large following of patients.

Two additional disadvantages in anesthesia have been seen by some. One of these arises from the belief that the anesthetist's activities are confined to the operating room, and the other is the conviction that a physician anesthetist is a technician doing work that could be done equally well by nurses. As in any type of work, the pattern of activity is cut by the individual concerned. A physician anesthetist can confine his work to the operating room, be seldom seen elsewhere in the hospital or in other medical activities and be compared properly with a technician. However, if he is a physician interested in his patients before, during and after anesthesia and conducts himself in a truly professional manner in and out of the operating room, neither of the above-mentioned thoughts will occur to him or to his associates.

The amount of training required to practice anesthesiology depends upon the type of practice in which one intends to engage. The American Board of anesthesiology requires two years of training in an approved residency program plus three additional years of practice in the specialty. There have been moves to increase the required residency training to three years, but this change has not yet materialized. Two years of residency training may be sufficient to provide the experience necessary to manage the majority of clinical anesthetic problems. However, for the physician who intends to deal with the specialized aspects of anesthesiology, to engage in teaching or in investigation, three or more years of training is preferable.

Certain characteristics of residency training in anesthesiology deserve mention. During the first year the trainee's attention is almost completely occupied with the acquisition of technical skills. There are many agents and many technics to be mastered. While there are certain similarities among them, there are also outstanding differences. The novice must learn to think and act simultaneously. He must learn the physical characteristics of the equipment he uses, to induce anesthesia smoothly and without the multitude of complications that occur commonly, to monitor the patient's vital signs, and to assess the patient's condition while attempting to judge the level of anesthesia (an all too difficult feat even for the accomplished anesthetist), and he must observe that the conditions provided for the surgeon are optimal. To do these things simultaneously is difficult enough, yet to do them with the knowledge that improperly treated complications may result in permanent damage to the patient, or an improperly assessed level of anesthesia may lead to death on the one hand or jeopardize the surgeon's performance on the other, poses distinct challenge. It is only after the development of a second sense permitting minute-to-minute appraisal of the proper level of anesthesia and the patient's condition that the trainee is able to turn his attention to other aspects of the specialty and to indulge in the individual interests that make anesthesiology so intriguing. The prerequisite of the early acquisition of technical skill in residency training is not unique to anesthesiology. The surgical resident must equally acquire technical skill during his training program.

An operating room is charged with the potential for emotional outbursts. Unexpected pathologic findings, unanticipated surgical and anesthetic complications, sudden hemorrhage, an unusually full operative schedule, inadequate surgical, anesthetic or nursing help, unexpected delays—all may lead to frayed tempers. This is understandable. Fortunately, pique is seldom carried beyond the door of the operating room. Yet such an atmosphere is not conducive to placing the neophyte at ease. One such emotional scene may make the beginner "gun shy" for weeks to come. Fortunately, there are fewer prima donnas in the operating room now, and with the passage of time nearly all may disappear from the scene. Nevertheless, the beginner should be aware that personal conflicts may occur and that during them the surgeon may be intolerant of inexperience.

Nor are patients usually aware of what constitutes the best in anesthetic practice. They may not realize or they may underestimate the hazard in being anesthetized. Their concerns relate principally to self-comfort and only secondarily to safety. They may not wish to remember the trip to the operating room; they usually dislike ether (all malodorous anesthetics are ether to them); they are convinced that nausea, vomiting and pain are inevitable, yet readily avoidable, postoperative sequelae. Compared with safety, these desires are trivial, but they can present an obstacle to the new anesthetist. Often he feels forced to order excessive preanesthetic medication or to avoid certain anesthetics solely to placate the patient. He may jeopardize safety in an attempt to provide comfort. The novice and his instructors must be aware of the problem constantly and must take appropriate measures to avoid the pitfalls.

There are three categories of practice in anesthesiology. These will be considered separately:

1. *Clinical Practice.* Most anesthesiologists are engaged solely or principally in clinical practice. These practices vary with the type of hospital wherein the practice is conducted. In small community institutions, anesthetic practice involves patients who are usually in good physical condition scheduled for relatively simple elective operations. Anesthesiologists work alone in these positions or have the assistance of one or more nurse technicians. Remuneration is usually on a fee for service basis with the patient reimbursing the physician directly. There are often significant advantages in living in small communities, but some have complained of intellectual isolation under these circumstances.

In larger hospitals the number of patients for surgical operations is greater, and the schedule may include all varieties of operations. Considerable time may be spent doing consultative work. In such locations anesthetists usually form groups so that an individual's work load is not excessive. There is an exchange of ideas, discussion of common problems and greater protection of time away from the hospital through the arrangement of call schedules. Many anesthesiologists in urban areas maintain private offices outside hospitals. Here patients are seen in consultation prior to admission to the hospital for surgical procedures or for diagnostic and therapeutic nerve blocks. A few offices are equipped with minor operating rooms and recovery rooms where surgeons and dentists can bring patients to be anesthetized for minor operative procedures on an out-patient basis.

2. *Clinical Practice With Teaching.* Teaching offers a challenge to the instructor to keep abreast of modern advances in his specialty and to understanding thoroughly the anesthetic technics and the actions of drugs he uses. Many find this stimulus invaluable. Clinical instruction lifts the most routine case out of the uninteresting and boring class into an invigorating experience. All types of clinical work are usually available in teaching practices, and many anesthesiologists devote a large amount of their time to individual interests such as the treatment of pain. In the large teaching centers a considerable proportion of the day must be devoted to other than clinical practice. Clinical instruction and supervision, lectures, demonstrations, conferences and seminars may occupy the major number of working hours. Income from patient care must often be supplemented from other sources.

3. *Clinical Practice With Teaching and Research.* This type of practice is most often associated with one of the major hospitals of the country or with medical schools. It varies little from that outlined above. The principal difference is the availability of the stimulus, the counsel and the facilities to carry on one or more research projects. These practices usually consist of a greater total daily work load, yet with less clinical work per individual. The nature of research projects varies from fundamental laboratory work to clinical investigation of new drugs. What can be accomplished in research in anesthesia is dependent only upon the training and the capa-

bilities of the anesthesiologist. Often association with basic science departments in medical schools enhances the research potential. One must perforce keep abreast of the newer advances of the specialty. One has the opportunity to attend meetings more regularly and is in a position to enjoy the privileges of academic life.

Few physicians are engaged in full-time or nearly full-time research in anesthesiology. Nevertheless, the demand for persons interested in and qualified for such positions is great, and the problems demanding solution are without limit. Many of the technics of investigation are those that would be used in the pharmacological or physiological laboratory and also in monitoring patients in the operating room. This increases the versatility of the investigator and enables him to take advantage of the many interesting situations that arise during operation. It also increases the opportunity for studies in patients to be anesthetized for surgical operations. Nearly all of the full-time investigators in anesthesiology are competent in laboratory as well as clinical investigation.

It is apparent from a consideration of the practices available that the prospective anesthesiologist has several situations from which to choose. In addition, the available positions are such that he is usually at liberty to select urban or rural, seacoast or plain location, and academic or clinical, group or individual practice. He should also consider that many practices are mixed. He may find it stimulating to do full-time clinical practice in a group where an active research practice exists.

Anesthesiology might be considered a bridge between the basic sciences and clinical medicine. Scarcely anywhere else in medicine are the fundamental principles of pharmacology and physiology so interwoven with the daily practice. This bridge will be strengthened and broadened, and even closer relations between basic scientists and clinicians can be anticipated. In many institutions, anesthesiologists do more to bring these groups together than do representatives of any other branch of medicine.

As mentioned earlier, the anesthesiologist must understand

the nature of the diseases that may be associated with surgical conditions. The number of patients in older age groups and those with complicating diseases of the brain, the heart and the lung is increasing. Their preparation for operation and their care during and after operation requires extraordinary skill, since the morbidity and the mortality of surgical patients is directly related to the age and the physical condition of the patient. Patients with complicating diseases challenge the anesthetist, and their survival from anesthesia and operation depends upon his skill. He must be familiar with the application of local and general anesthetics, vasopressor agents, analgesic drugs, and cerebral and cardiac stimulant drugs in a large number of internal diseases. He must be able to interpret correctly the electrocardiogram and the electroencephalogram. He has been called by some "the internist of the operating room." His training has made him invaluable in the diagnosis and the treatment of acute medical and surgical emergencies. The anesthesiologist will assume an increasingly important role in the care of patients in the hospital and in the general training of interns and medical students. As our population continues to age, the demand for anesthesiologists must become greater.

The last decade has seen a tremendous step forward in attempts to ensure patient safety during anesthesia and operation by the use of monitoring devices. In most institutions, the anesthesia department supervises these instruments and is responsible for their correct interpretation. Much of this equipment has been developed through the co-ordinated activities of anesthetists and electronic engineers. There is little question that further strides will be taken, that there will be more universal application of monitoring devices, and that new and useful physiological and pharmacological data will be accumulated. Few other fields have so much to offer the physician with an orientation in electronics.

The field of research as applied to anesthesiology is unlimited. No one has yet explained the basis for narcosis. While it is unlikely that the explanation will come from the operating room or from man as the subject, nevertheless significant observations in this direction can be made on patients. The perfect anesthetic has not yet been discovered. The projects that await solution in the interrelated fields of anesthesiology and the physiology and the pharmacology of respiration, circulation, bodily metabolism and the central nervous, endocrine and muscular systems are great in number. The missing item is a sufficient number of interested persons with adequate background to accomplish the tasks.

BIBLIOGRAPHY

Betcher, A. M., Ciliberti, B. J., Wood, P. M., and Wright, L. H.: The jubilee year of organized anesthesia, Anesthesiology *17*:226-264, 1956.

Bonica, J. J.: The Management of Pain, Philadelphia, Lea & Febiger, 1953.

Cullen, S. C.: Attitudes and practices, Anesthesiology *21*:322-323, 1960.

Dornette, W. H. L., and Brechner, V. L.: Instrumentation in Anesthesiology, Philadelphia, Lea & Febiger, 1959.

Foldes, F. F.: Muscle Relaxants in Anesthesiology, Springfield, Ill., Thomas, 1957.

Moore, D. C.: Regional Block, Springfield, Ill., Thomas, 1953.

Safar, P., and McMahon, M.: Mouth-to-airway emergency artificial respiration, J.A.M.A. *166*:1459, 1958.

Wigodsky, H. S.: Anesthesiologists—today and tomorrow, Anesthesiology *21*:78-81, 1960.

HARRIET L. HARDY, M.D.

Assistant Medical Director, Chief of the Occupational Medical Service, Massachusetts Institute of Technology; Lecturer on Medicine, Harvard Medical School

17

Occupational Medicine

With some justice, medical practitioners have been accused of lack of interest in affairs outside the limits of their discipline. It is true that the urgent demands of active clinical medicine absorb the attention and the energy of the conscientious physician. And satisfaction derived from the healing arts is often great enough to preclude interest in other professions, political affairs and economic changes. Occupational health, by its content and point of view, provides a professional life for the physician that makes it possible for him to be an active member of our industrial, social and even political life.

It is against the background of the many changes begun by the Industrial Revolution and violently accelerated by wars, atomic energy development, world-wide communication and expanding technologic demands that the physician, planning his future, may want to consider the field of occupational health. In many ways, this field is not a specialty but rather a point of view for a well-trained physician. "Occupational medicine" is a term that is preferred to the often-used title of industrial medicine to describe the care of workers with job-related accidents or disease. The word "occupational" broadens the title of this field of medicine to include research workers, farmers, executives, in addition to groups of men and women engaged in factory work such as textile manufacture, or heavy labor such as underground mining. With the increase in prosperity in the United States and the health consciousness of workers and their union leaders, as well as the vision of public health leaders of promoting good health, an even broader concept is emerging. The term "occupational health" is used to convey this increasingly popular concept of the doctor's efforts aimed toward protecting and increasing the general well-being of the working population. Government agencies charged with guarding the health and the safety of industrial workers, certain insurance companies and some large industries describe the technical preventive aspects of their work in this field as occupational or industrial hygiene. Occupational hygienists may be engineers, physicists or chemists trained to use their skills in the prevention of job-related illness by control of potentially harmful work exposures.

Before presenting the current prospect for a physician considering a career in occupational health, certain high points of the history of this specialty here and abroad will illustrate the unusual tradition in this field.

There are records in ancient Egyptian inscriptions dated about 2300 B.C. of not only palace and tomb physicians but also physicians whose duty was the care of underground mine workers. Hunter suggests that in ancient cultures and all through the Dark Ages the diseases of workers were neglected because of class distinctions, the health of slaves and uneducated workmen being no concern of the rich and the privileged. Alice Hamilton writes that in Roman times mercury poisoning was a disease of slaves. Plutarch, in the first century A.D., blamed a mine owner as unjust because he used slaves who were not also criminals.

In 1556 Agricola, a German, wrote of the lung diseases of metal miners in Central Europe as follows: "If the dust has corrosive qualities, it eats away the lungs, and implants consumption in the body. In the mines of the Carpathian Mountains women are found who have married seven husbands, all of whom this terrible consumption has carried off to a premature death." This reflects the well-known observation that dust in the lungs predisposes to a fulminating form of tuberculosis. Another extraordinary physician of the 16th century, Paracelsus, wrote with great accuracy of the diseases of smelter workers and metallurgists. He described faithfully the symptoms of acute and chronic mercury poisoning.

In 1713 Ramazzini wrote his famous book *De Morbis Artificum Diatriba* describing the potential hazards of 52 occupations, among them wrestling, grave-digging, nursing. This established him as the father of occupational health. Ramazzini, in referring to the writings of Hippocrates, who described so well how to take a good medical history, suggested that he should have added one more question to his list and asked the patient to describe his occupation.

James Watt's invention of the steam engine in 1769 marks the beginning of the Industrial Revolution which completely changed the life of those countries that embraced the resulting technologic advances. The great social changes surrounding urbanization and industrialization brought great riches to a few and great misery to many. English writers of the early 19th century, among them Blake, Dickens and Lamb, described dramatically the resulting social and economic problems. Until the work of Charles Thackrah (1795-1832) physicians seem to have ignored the many diseases brought about by the conditions of industrial life. Thackrah wrote as follows in 1831: "Myself and my pupils have personally and carefully inspected the state of the artisans in most kinds of manufacture, examined the agencies believed to be injurious, conversed on the subjects with masters, overlookers, and the more intelligent workmen, and obtained many tables illustrating the characters of the disorders prevalent in the several kinds of employ. . . . From a reference to fact and observations . . . in many of our occupations, the injurious agents might be immediately removed or diminished. Evils are suffered to exist, even when the means of correction are known and easily applied. Thoughtlessness or apathy is the only obstacle to success." This last observation is extraordinarily apt today.

There are exceptions to the general statement that the medical profession was unaware of the harmful environmental insults to the 19th century workers. A dramatic example is provided by Sir Percival Potts' description of carcinoma of the scrotum occurring in chimney sweeps in London. These poor boys, under 10 years of age, were forced in and out of chimney pots, rubbing carcinogenic materials from domestic soot into their filthy clothes which, since they were rarely changed, acted to keep the dangerous chemical in close contact with the scrotal sac. However, the literary men were on the whole more interested in these man-made problems than many physicians. In 1863 in his *Water Babies,* Charles Kingsley wrote of his main character, Tom, a chimney sweep: "Once upon a time there was a little chimney-sweep, and his name was Tom. He cried half his life, and laughed the other half. He cried when he had to climb the dark flues, rubbing his poor knees and elbows raw; and when the soot got into his eyes, which it did every day in the week; and when he had not enough to eat, which happened every day in the week likewise."

Great social reforms, backed by legislation, took place in Europe during the latter half of the 19th century and continue into the 20th century, constantly aiming to correct hazardous working conditions or to compensate, however poorly, the injured workman and his family.

Because the United States was an agricultural country until after the war of 1812, our history relevant to occupational health is a little different. Not until 1820 were textile mills or metal and coal mining established industries, in which increasingly varied technical demands produced needed mechanics and master craftsmen. Beginning about this time and continuing to the present, immigrants came from many lands to work as cheap labor, especially in building roads and railroads, in lumbering, and eventually to be employed in all industry throughout the country. These workers, usually ignorant, accepted a poor working environment and low wages. However, the first labor movement in this country began in the late 1820's and is credited with achieving suffrage for all men, public school education, and control of the length of the working day. In this industrial picture physicians were needed, but there is very little evidence of professional interest until the second decade of the 20th century. Dr. Benjamin W. McCready, later one of the founders of the Bellevue Hospital Medical College, wrote in 1837 the winning essay in competition for a prize offered by the New York State Medical Society entitled "On the Influence of Trades, Professions, and Occupations in the United States in the Production of Disease"; this was the first recognized medical writing on this subject. He found difficulty collecting knowledge on the subject and says that he rarely got answers from those "most competent to pronounce upon the questions," and what information he got from those in authority was often contradictory. McCready talked with workmen and reports them "so little attentive to the causes which affect their health, and their views are so often warped by prejudice or interest, that little reliance can be placed upon them." These comments could refer to current conditions in some parts of the country. The essay is most interesting and develops considerable data on the hazards and the hardships of the work of his day with long passages on improvement in health to be gained by proper food, rest, exercise, recreation and good housing. Under the heading "artizans," McCready describes among others the problems and the advantages of the work of tailors, shoemakers, butchers, carvers, coopers, painters. For example, McCready reports that tailors are short-lived, suffer from poor digestion, drink excessively, develop phthisis readily, have a two-inch less measurement around the chest than the average artisan. In contrast, "coopers have sufficient exercise, and are not subject to dust or other noxious agents. The employment is healthy." A few sentences from the description of the dangers to seamstresses reflects McCready's broad interests in his patients' occupations.

"There is one source of ill-health affecting a portion of this class of persons (the seamstresses) which, from its nature, must be touched upon with peculiar delicacy. After working during the whole day, if per chance they have an evening to spare, instead of employing it in a manner calculated to invigorate their enfeebled habits, they hurry off to a prayer-meeting or a lecture, where, in a crowded and ill-ventilated room, they are exposed to sources of excitement, which the already exalted sensibility of their nervous system renders doubly injurious. On Sunday, too, not contented with attending church three times a day, many of them are likewise engaged for several hours in the Sabbath schools. Such a line of conduct is almost sure to break down a constitution originally feeble."

There are only scattered writings on occupational medical subjects until 1914 when W. G. Thompson, Professor of Medicine at Cornell University, published a comprehensive textbook entitled *The Occupational Diseases: Their Causation, Symptoms, Treatment, and Prevention*. This book (704 pages of information, much of it applicable today) accomplished what the author describes in the preface: "This work, which is the first of its kind to be published in this country, is designed primarily for physicians interested in the subject of the Occupational Diseases of Modern Life, and also as a guide for students of social economics, social service workers, insurance actuaries, and those whose special interests deal with problems of labor legislation, or with workers in the chemical, textile, and many other manufactures or trades in which the health of the workman is closely related to problems of efficiency and humanitarian efforts."

The United States lagged behind Europe in legislation to control harmful working conditions, and far behind the rest of the world with respect to the attention paid by physicians to the effects of toxic materials. Only a few individuals were deeply interested, but they stimulated government and labor organizations between 1907 and 1920 to take action. Dr. W. G. Thompson and Dr. Alice Hamilton stand out as students and writers in this field who made such personal and professional contributions that when the great depression and the World Wars brought inevitable social changes, a solid though modest tradition in the field of occupational health was already established. A few quotations from Dr. Hamilton's autobiography

(*Exploring Dangerous Trades*) makes this period vivid. In 1910 Dr. Hamilton visited Brussels to attend the Fourth International Congress on Occupational Accidents and Diseases. She writes as follows: "The Brussels Congress was a very interesting experience for me, meeting and hearing the famous authorities I knew so well from their writings: chiefly German and English, but also French, Austrian, Dutch, Belgian, Italian. But for an American it was not an occasion for national pride. There were but two of us on the program, Major Bailey Ashford, with a paper on hookworm infestation in Puerto Rico, and myself with one on the white-lead industry in the United States which revealed only too clearly the lack of such precautions as were a commonplace in the older countries. It was still more mortifying to be unable to answer any of the questions put to us: What was the rate of lead poisoning in such and such an industry? What legal regulations did we have for the dangerous trades? What was the system of compensation? Finally Dr. Glibert, of the Belgian Labor Department, dismissed the subject: 'It is well known that there is no industrial hygiene in the United States. Ça n'existe pas.' . . .

"American medical authorities had never taken industrial diseases seriously, the American Medical Association had never held a meeting on the subject, and while European journals were full of articles on industrial poisoning, the number published in American medical journals up to 1910 could be counted on one's fingers. . . .

"When I talked to my medical friends about the strange silence on this subject in American medical magazines and textbooks, I gained the impression that here was a subject tainted with Socialism or with feminine sentimentality for the poor. . . . Everyone with whom I talked assured me that the foreign writings could not apply to American conditions, for our workmen were so much better paid, their standard of living was so much higher, and the factories they worked in so much finer in every way than the European, that they did not suffer from the evils to which the poor foreign was subject. That sort of talk always left me skeptical. And presently I had factual confirmation of my disbelief in the happy lot of the American worker through the reading of John Andres' manuscript on 'phossy jaw' in the match industry in the United States. . . . Sometimes the abscess forms in the upper jaw and works up into the orbit, causing the loss of an eye. In severe cases one lower jawbone may have to be removed. . . . There are cases on record of men and women who had to live all the rest of their days on liquid food. The scars and contractures left after recovery were terribly disfiguring, and led some women to commit suicide. Here was an industrial disease which could be clearly demonstrated to the most skeptical."

This record of lack of responsibility for worker health has been changing steadily since the middle '20's. Some industries have had excellent medical and engineering advice to control hazardous jobs for years. Individual physicians and investigators have become interested in industrial diseases, contributing by their efforts to the care of workers and to understanding of the behavior of toxic materials in the body. Aub's work on lead poisoning and Martland's contribution in the study of radium-induced damage are outstanding examples of studies whose influence is still in effect in prevention and handling of certain industrial disease. Legislation and the efforts of organized labor have forced reluctant industries to take steps to control hazardous work. Workmen's compensation laws and health and safety laws of Labor Departments vary from state to state, but in general by economic pressure they have caused great improvements in working conditions throughout the United States. Added to such evolutionary social and economic pressures are the rapid advances in our prosperity, the consequent demands both for labor and goods, and more recently the unpredictable needs of our military services. Thus it is that occupational health has become a very important and expanding field that will require more and more medical manpower.

These illustrative bits of the history of occupational medicine in the past bring out the fact that until recently only a few well-trained physicians have sensed the rich opportunity offered by this field of interest. According to McCord, in 1912 in the United States there were "scarcely more than a score" of doctors who organized the American Association of Industrial Physicians and Surgeons. The majority of these were trained in traumatic surgery and did little in any other branch of occupational health except to advise the management of the industry they served. At present there are about 4000 members of the Industrial Medical Association, an organization which, while not including all physicians is representative of the great growth of the field of occupational health into all medical specialties. In 1949, the American Academy of Occupational Medicine was formed with the purpose of setting high standards of training and performance and attracting well-trained doctors on a full-time basis. The present membership of the Academy is 300, proof of the fact that occupational health is an attractive specialty. A final step in recognizing occupational medicine as a specialty was realized in 1955, when the American Board of Preventive Medicine established certification for membership to well-trained physicians practicing occupational health. The requirements for certification are as follows:

1. Successful completion (after internship) of at least two academic years of graduate study in preventive and occupational medicine in a school of medicine, or a school of public health. The schools in which such instruction is provided shall be accredited for graduate study by the Council on Medical Education and Hospitals of the American Medical Association or the American Public Health Association, in accordance with the jurisdictions of these accrediting agencies; or training and study deemed by the Board to be substantially equivalent to such graduate study.

2. Completion (after internship) of not less than one year, in addition to 1 above, of supervised experience (residency) in occupational medical practice in an industrial or medical organization. This residency shall provide planned instruction, observation and active participation in a comprehensive program of occupational

medicine; or a comparable period of experience deemed by the Board to be substantially equivalent to such year of supervised experience.

3. A period (after internship) of not less than three years, in addition to 1 and 2 above, of special training in, or teaching or practice of, occupational medicine.

4. Limitation of practice to full-time teaching, research, or practice of occupational medicine.

The field of occupational health is thus demonstrated to be growing and changing with the rush of technical advances and political pressures so insistent currently. However, to be specific, what are the various positions that a physician may consider within this specialty?

The full-time plant physician is in great demand at present. Many companies, either because they sense the value of promoting the health of their workers or because of pressure from unions and liability insurance companies, insist on obtaining sound medical and industrial hygiene advice. The character of the physicians' work varies with the industry. For example, operations using chemicals, smelting operations and nuclear reactors for power production each present unique problems which differ completely from those of large department stores and utility companies with many clerical helpers. Pioneer work remains to be done in many positions in industry. In many instances an industry has never had medical help, and its president has only the knowledge of the care of his own illness or that of his family in judging medical competence. In addition, the character of occupational hazards to health changes very rapidly with our advancing technology. Medical knowledge available for diagnosis and handling of occupational illness also adds to the interest and the satisfaction of the practitioner. As Kammer, Head of the Department of Occupational Health at the University of Pittsburgh puts it, the full-time successful practitioner in this field must be in the position of saying "that he has mastery over the most advanced technologies thus far devised: modern industry and modern health sciences."

The full-time industrial doctor must also like his fellow

man because he often has to "sell" good medical practice even to those who pay his wages. His daily round finds him advising or being advised by many nonmedical colleagues such as the safety engineer, the production manager, the industrial hygienist, the company or insurance company lawyer, and the union steward. The common purpose is to ensure and promote the health of the workers in his charge. Great skill and tact are required for the physician working for and with the industry while preserving the privacy of relations with his patients.

Another choice of a career in occupational health is offered by the increasing number of government agencies that have positions for physicians interested in the study and the control of environmental disease. The federal public health service, the state, and a few city public health and labor departments, the Atomic Energy Commission, all branches of the military services employ at present physicians for a variety of jobs. The need for them is on the increase. Underwater diving in nuclear-powered submarines, outer space exploration by humans, exposure to previously unknown energies in atomic energy development are examples of present problems requiring both basic and animal research. Because of the urgency of some of these problems, immediate imaginative planning on the basis of presently known physiologic responses must be translated into action. The older problems of lead poisoning, pulmonary dust disease, hepatic and hematologic disease from exposure to solvents remain as a challenge both to the research worker and the physician dedicated to the prevention of manmade disease. Skills of the epidemiologist, the occupational hygiene engineer and chemist, the biostatistician come into play in a community or an industry when an unusual incidence of disease appears to be job related. The government agency, acting to advise industrial management, worker and medical practitioner may play an exciting role as, for example, in relating neighborhood cases of beryllium poisoning to uncontrolled release of toxic beryllium compounds from beryllium extraction operations. The rapidly mounting lay and professional interest in relating atmospheric pollution to the occurrence of pulmonary malignancy is a new challenge to government activity in the field of occupational health. A colleague, Christine Einert, working in the field within a governmental agency writes that occupational medicine lacks routine predictable duties and is more concerned with helping people than producing a cure of a single person. Further, the practitioner in this field must be interested in unsolved medical problems and be happy to work with colleagues who are disciplined in both the physical sciences and sociology. Perhaps most basic of all to the medical student in considering work in occupational health both in industry and government agencies is the concept of health as not merely the absence of disease. Real satisfaction comes both to the laboratory worker and to the practitioner who strives to keep well people well and ideally even to improve the state of health.

There is a serious shortage of well-qualified physicians for smaller industrial concerns. Shepard reports than 99 per cent of all employers in the United States have fewer than 500 on their payroll, with the result that of 50,000,000 workers few will have medical advice on the job. Depending on the size and the industrial character of the community in which the young practitioner finds himself, he may consider serving one or more small industries. In this situation there are dangers to both industry and the physician, especially if the latter is building a private practice. One student of this problem writes "the arrangement is started with some semblance of good intentions on the part of the physician, particularly when he is a young man beginning practice. As time goes on the demands of private practice encroach successfully upon the responsibilities at the plant: the physician arrives late and he leaves early, and finally he is carrying on his practice over the telephone during the short time he is actually in the plant." On the other hand, the doctor who sees the rewards already outlined in this field of preventive medicine will also see the wisdom of arranging his program to suit the needs of the industry. Kehoe writes vigorously of what must be done: "A great opportunity is now open to the medical profession, in that almost any contribution made by it toward the solution of the obvious hygienic problems of industry will demonstrate the profession's usefulness to society. This is even more significant because the employees of small industrial plants represent more than half of our total industrial population. Professional responsibility and prestige demand that the attention of physicians and medical educators be directed toward the problems of human health that derive from the most characteristic and insistent activity of modern life—technological industrial production. The productive functioning of this segment of our population, impaired as it is by the inroads of preventable disability and absenteeism, is a matter of great economic and social importance."

The catalogue of prospects in this field includes several more professional paths. There are a few well-qualified internists in this country who have become full-time private consultants with occupational disease as their sole interest. Such a course would follow academic training and experience in a government agency, in an industry, or after association with a well-established occupational medical consultant. The fascination in this possibility lies in working on diagnostic problems and planning preventive measures for potentially dangerous work.

A number of universities, the National Institutes of Health, the U. S. Public Health Service, and industrially supported organizations encourage or undertake basic and applied research directed toward understanding the biologic behavior of chemicals, dusts, and physical energies at potentially harmful levels. Certain man-made diseases, by mimicking diseases of unknown cause, provide cludes for relevant investigation. As an example, after World War I malignancies of the bladder have been correlated with exposure to certain aniline derivatives, and a wealth of knowledge of some carcinogens has resulted. Beryllium disease is so very like sarcoidosis in clinical behavior, x-ray pattern and histopathologic picture that studies in pathogenesis of both diseases are stimulated. Research in the field of genetics is currently very active because of the need to know the safe levels of ionizing radiation to which workers may be exposed in atomic energy development.

Finally, the demands described for medical manpower in industry have resulted in the development of teaching departments for this purpose in a number of universities. Several departments doing teaching and research in occupational health are more than twenty-five years old; but the majority of the departments, chiefly in Schools of Public Health, date from the end of World War II. For the physician looking into the future of occupational health, consideration of two years of postdoctoral training, a period of practice of occupational medicine in industry for a period of years to be followed by teaching with or without investigative work provides a wonderfully interesting and rewarding professional life. An important variant of this kind of career is available and will become more so to the clinically trained physician who becomes interested in occupational medicine. Because medical schools do not, and perhaps cannot, include occupational health in the undergraduate medical curriculum, the medical education of the hospital resident may profitably include solid training in job-related disease. The internist alert to environmental etiology, who preferably has first-hand knowledge of industry, is ideally suited to handle bedside and clinic teaching in the diagnosis and the handling of occupational illness. While there are not at present established posts for such teaching, the demand is being felt.

The doctor who chooses a career in occupational health will by necessity learn many new and strange facets of other disciplines. He will be extraordinarily useful to our society through the prevention of illness and through the establishment of conditions favorable to good health, be he practitioner, teacher, or investigator. The personal satisfaction derived from using one's professional training to be a part of the changes of one's times can hardly be exaggerated.

BIBLIOGRAPHY

Aub, Joseph C., Fairhall, L. T., Minot, A. S., and Reznikoff, P.: Lead poisoning, Medicine 4:1, 1925.

Einert, Christine: Personal communication, July, 1960.

Hamilton, Alice: Exploring the Dangerous Trades, Boston, Little, Brown & Company, 1943.

Hamilton, Alice, and Hardy, Harriet L.: Industrial Toxicology, ed. 2, p. 104, New York, Hoeber, 1949.

Hunter, Donald: The Diseases of Occupations, Boston, Little, Brown & Company, 1955.

Kammer, A. G.: Personal communication, May, 1960.

Kehoe, Robert A.: Council on Industrial Health, J.A.M.A. 152:1262, 1953.

Martland, Harrison S.: Occupational poisoning in manufacture of luminous watch dials, J.A.M.A. 92:466, 552, 1929.

McCord, Carey P.: A Blind Hog's Acorns—Vignettes of the Maladies of Workers, New York, Cloud, Inc., 1945.

McCready, Benjamin W.: On the Influence of Trades, Professions, and Occupations in the United States, in the Production of Disease, pp. 1-31, 68-69, 87, Baltimore, Johns Hopkins Press, 1943.

Shepard, William P.: The practice of industrial medicine—what it takes, Journal of Occupational Medicine, 2:255, 1960.

Thompson, W. Gilman: The Occupational Diseases: Their Causation, Symptoms, Treatment and Prevention, New York, Appleton, 1914. (Preface.)

HOWARD A. RUSK, M.D.
*Professor of Physical Medicine and Rehabilitation
at New York University*

18

Physical Medicine and Rehabilitation

One of the greatest advances that has been made by medicine and surgery in the past two decades is the new acceptance of a third dimension of medical and surgical responsibility—rehabilitation.

Physical medicine and rehabilitation offers some of the oldest therapeutic tools known to medicine, yet it is one of the newest medical specialties. It has often been termed the "third phase of medicine" following "preventive medicine" and "curative medicine and surgery." It is that period when the "fever is down and the stitches are out," the period "between the bed and the job." In contrast with "convalescence," in which the patient is left alone to let nature and time take their course, rehabilitation is a dynamic concept in which the skills of the rehabilitation team, consisting of the physician, physical therapists, occupational therapists, nurses, social workers, counselors and other trained personnel, are integrated as a single force to assist the patient in reaching the maximum of his physical, emotional and social and vocational potentials.

The first objective of rehabilitation is to eliminate the physical disability if that is possible; the second, to reduce or alleviate the disability to the greatest extent possible; and the third, to retrain the person with a residual physical disability "to live and to work within the limits of his disability but to the hilt of his capabilities."

Effective rehabilitation depends upon the skills and the services of members of many professions. However, the physician, by the very nature of the problem, must be the leader of the team. Fundamental to the effectiveness of all the component disciplines of rehabilitation is the adequacy of medical services (for in practically all instances, the other component services are based upon the degree of severity of the residual physical disability, which cannot be eliminated or further reduced by medical services). If self-sufficiency in job placement or adequacy of self-care is the end objective of rehabilitation, certainly rehabilitation-oriented medical care starting at the earliest possible moment following acute illness or injury is the foundation.

Until the last 50 years, the saving of human life as the traditional and cherished goal of medicine was largely a matter of saving individual patients. With the first half of the 20th century, the whole character of medicine's traditional goal was changed. The expansion of research into the etiology and the therapy of communicable and infectious diseases "struck specifics."

The establishment of new and effective public health measures and some of the rich findings in the basic science fields reported earlier in this book gave the life-saving functions of medicine mass proportions. These, combined with similar advances in the greater availability of medical and hospital care, improved nutrition, increased education, better housing and all the contributing factors to our unprecedented current standard of living, mean that hundreds of thousands of persons are alive today who at the turn of the century would have died with the same medical problems.

Yet many of them have not come out unscathed. They have survived only to find themselves confronted with residual disability. The paraplegic whose back is broken in a fall does not die today as he would have done 50 years ago. He has strong arms, an active mind and a burning desire to live the best life he can with what he has left. Antibiotics control the upper respiratory and urinary tract infections of the severely involved cerebral palsied youngster who would have succumbed before their development. He seeks his place in society. The survivors of infection get their share of the degenerative diseases. These are present-day problems that must be solved.

The day-to-day experience of all practicing physicians shows that not only has there been a substantial increase in the gross number of disabled persons, but that a growing percentage of our population suffers from long-term illnesses and substantial physical impairments. Two thousand years ago the average length of life was only 25 years; at the turn of the century, it was 49; by 1950 it had reached 67; and we are now on the threshold of the Biblical three score and ten. Contrary to opinions expressed by some, the growing incidence of chronic disability is a tribute to medicine rather than an indictment of it. But as the physician has been largely responsible for this development, he must assume leadership in its solution.

Until recent years, the great majority of the medical profession looked upon rehabilitation as an extracurricular activity of medicine: something dealing with social work and vocational training, but something that had little concern and held but few implications for medicine. Today, however, that trend is being reversed and, although there are still many physicians who are unfamiliar with the aims and the procedures of rehabilitation, more and more is medicine beginning to recognize that medical care cannot be considered complete until the patient with a residual physical disability has been trained "to live and work with what he has left." Except in a few isolated instances, the physically handicapped person must be retrained to walk and travel, to care for his daily needs, to use normal methods of transportation, to use ordinary toilet facilities, to apply and remove his own prosthetic devices and to communicate either orally or in writing. These are such simple things that they are often overlooked, but the personal, vocational and social success of the handicapped person is dependent upon them.

Experience has shown that if the practitioner or specialist responsible for the patient's primary medical care will take the necessary time, he can provide the necessary rehabilitation services for most patients. This is as it should be, for such services should be an integral part of basic medical and surgical care.

However, there are a number of patients with severe disabilities—paraplegia, quadriplegia, hemiplegia with aphasia, the demyelinating diseases—whose needs cannot be met without a concentrated long-term program that includes full utilization of all the ancillary medical disciplines and specialized rehabilitation technics. It is obvious that no medical practitioner, general or specialist, can have at his disposal for the care of his patients all of the varied facilities, equipment, specialized skills and ancillary medical personnel needed for the management of such patients. The answer, as has been traditional in the development of all medical specialties, is the provision of opportunities for physicians to acquire these specialized skills.

Specialty certification by the American Board of Physical Medicine and Rehabilitation has among its requirements three years of residency training in an approved hospital residency training program. A year of residency training in internal medicine, pediatrics, neurology or orthopedic surgery can be substituted for one of these three years. Currently, in 1960, there are 64 institutions that have approved three-year residencies in physical medicine and rehabilitation. These are primary residencies and this figure does not include the separate hospitals that may be utilized to make up a single residency program. These training programs can accommodate a total of approximately 260 residents.

At present there are only approximately 350 board-certified specialists in physical medicine and rehabilitation in the United States. Because of the great national shortage of such specialists, the Federal Government, through the Office of

Vocational Rehabilitation of the Department of Health, Education and Welfare, is now providing fellowships* to physicians who wish to take postgraduate training in physical medicine and rehabilitation.

Although a number of specialists in physical medicine and rehabilitation are engaged in private practice and maintain offices for this purpose, most are also members of the staff of one or more hospitals or rehabilitation centers. In some instances, hospital services are limited to a physical medicine and rehabilitation unit, which accepts in-patients and out-patients through referral for evaluation and treatment, but there is a growing trend for hospitals to establish physical medicine and rehabilitation services as major services with an allocation of beds. When such services are established, the physical medicine and rehabilitation service functions as a "service" to the other units of the hospital much in the same manner as the x-ray and laboratory units.

At New York City's Bellevue Hospital, for example, the rehabilitation service that was founded in 1946 as the first such service in any civilian general hospital in the world provides consultants for each of the other major services such as fracture, pediatrics, orthopedics, surgery and neurology. Its resident and visiting staff regularly makes rounds with the resident and visiting staff of these services. For example, its staff may see a patient in consultation before his leg is removed, indoctrinating him in what he must expect, why he cannot keep his stump on a pillow, why he has to lie on his abdomen. Of course, medical responsibility during the period of definitive care rests with the initial or admitting service. As soon as the stitches are removed, the patient is transferred to a rehabilitation ward. At this time, the rehabilitation service assumes the major responsibility for his care, including fitting of the prosthesis and training in its uses. The roles are now reversed; the surgical service has become the consulting service.

----

* Information concerning fellowships in physical medicine and rehabilitation can be obtained from the Office of Vocational Rehabilitation, Department of Health, Education and Welfare, Washington 25, D. C.

However, before the actual transfer of the patient to a rehabilitation ward, he attends one of the rehabilitation service's semiweekly evaluation clinics, where his problem is analyzed and discussed by all members of the staff—physical therapists, occupational therapists, nurses, vocational counselors, speech therapists, social workers and psychologists—as well as resident and visiting medical staff. The decision as to the feasibility of transferring the patient to the rehabilitation service is then made on the basis of the service's ability to contribute to his over-all physical, emotional, social and vocational rehabilitation.

To ignore the development of rehabilitation services within general hospitals is to guarantee the continued deterioration of many less severely disabled persons until they, too, reach the severely disabled and totally dependent category. The neglect of disability is far more costly than an early aggressive program of rehabilitation that restores the individual to the highest possible level of physical, economic, social and emotional self-sufficiency.

Unfortunately, in the past, the medical attitude toward the chronically disabled has too often been one of hopelessness and passive acceptance. Experience with modern dynamic rehabilitation using the team approach has shown that much can be done to help these patients.

Hemiplegic patients, for example, have filled the back beds of our medical wards and the back bedrooms of their families' homes and have crowded the few available beds in nursing homes and institutions for the chronically disabled. However, studies have shown that 90 per cent of all hemiplegic patients can be taught ambulation, self-care and urinary and fecal continence; 50 per cent can be taught to do gainful work.

More recent studies have also indicated that there is no correlation between the degree of the neurologic insult and success in rehabilitation. The three most important questions in the rehabilitation of the hemiplegic patient are: (1) does he have a job to which he can go, (2) does he have a home and (3) does someone love him?

As in all great social movements, the increased interest in rehabilitation during the past two decades has been a result of the impact and the recognition of increased needs—in this instance, the rapid increase in the developed parts of the world of the incidence of chronic disability as a result of the increasing age of the population.

Although some nations of the world still have pressing problems of communicable disease, and life-expectancy rates vary from nation to nation, depending on the availability of medical care, public health measures, food supply and the general standard of living, the trend in all nations is toward a greatly increased life expectancy, with the result that throughout the world the population is gradually becoming older.

At the same time that the average age is advancing in the developed parts of the world, a new concept of the dignity of man and the value of the worth of the individual is beginning to emerge in those nations of the world that do not have the benefits as yet of modern programs of public health and medical care. This new concept of the worth of the individual has been symbolized and is finding its expression in many cases in the desire of these nations to institute programs of services for their physically handicapped.

It is essential that any physician considering entering physical medicine and rehabilitation as a career share this new concept of the worth of the individual. The rewards that come to the physiatrist are not the immediate satisfactions that come from a successful diagnosis of a complex problem or the dramatic changes that result from surgery.

The personal satisfactions for the physiatrist come slowly. Many of his more severely disabled patients have long-standing disabilities. Progress with them is frequently slow, and often little day-to-day change is seen. But he will have the warm glow of inner satisfaction from knowing that he is helping his fellow men to live rich and full lives despite their physical disabilities. To many of us, perhaps to you, this is important.

The prime requisite for success in physical medicine and

rehabilitation is the personality of the practitioner. He must, above all else, be a socially minded individual with a sincere desire to help others. But along with this personal trait, he must also enjoy working with people.

The number and the degree of interpersonal relations of the physiatrist is greater than that of any other specialist. First, he personally spends a great deal of time with the patient and his family. Second, he is the leader of a team of paramedical workers such as physical therapists, occupational therapists, speech and hearing therapists, social workers, rehabilitation counselors, psychologists, nurses, prosthetists and orthotists. Third, his work is entirely by referral, and he must maintain close contact with the physicians who refer patients to him, for they bear the primary medical responsibility for the over-all care of the patient. Fourth, the nature of the physiatrist's practice requires close co-operation with a variety of other specialists, such as internists, orthopedic surgeons, neurologists, neurosurgeons and urologists. In all of these interpersonal relations the physiatrist must have the earned respect and confidence of those with whom he works.

Rehabilitation during the first quarter of this century was characterized by the development of orthopedic surgery, physical therapy, occupational therapy and the State-Federal vocational rehabilitation program. All were direct outgrowths of World War I. Under the stimulus of World War II, the second quarter of the century has seen a recognition that the problems that medicine faces in meeting the growing incidence of chronic disease and disability extend far beyond any medical specialty; they are problems that must be faced and solved by medicine as a whole. The concept of rehabilitation and the basic technics must be made a part of the armamentarium of all physicians; for regardless of the type of disability, the responsibility of the physician to his patient cannot end when the acute injury or illness has been cared for. Medical care is not complete until the patient has been trained to live and to work with what he has left.

If any major attack is to be made on the problems of chronic disability, the general hospital and the individual practicing physician must be the focal points of that attack. It is only in doctors' offices and in general hospitals that such services can be brought to the patient at the earliest possible time and that the costly and damaging physical, emotional, social and vocational sequelae of the acute disease process or trauma may be alleviated or minimized.

Rehabilitation of the chronically ill and the chronically disabled is not just a series of restorative technics; it is a philosophy of medical responsibility. Failure to assume this responsibility means to guarantee the continued deterioration of many less severely disabled persons until they, too, reach the severely disabled and totally dependent category. The neglect of disability in its early stages is far more costly than an early aggressive program of rehabilitation that restores the individual to the highest possible level of physical, economic, social and emotional self-sufficiency.

BIBLIOGRAPHY

Allen, W. S.: Rehabilitation: A Community Challenge, New York, Wiley, 1958.

Covalt, D. A., *et al.*: Rehabilitation in Industry, New York, Grune & Stratton, 1958.

Kessler, H. H.: Rehabilitation of the Physically Handicapped, New York, Columbia Univ. Press, 1953.

Lowman, E. A.: Arthritis: General Principles of Physical Medicine and Rehabilitation, Boston, Little, 1959.

Rusk, H. A., *et al.*: Rehabilitation Medicine, St. Louis, Mosby, 1956.

LEONA BAUMGARTNER, M.D.

Professor of Public Health and Preventive Medicine at Cornell, and Commissioner of Health, City of New York

and

ROBERT E. ROTHERMEL, M.D.

Director of Professional Education, New York City Department of Health

19

Administration and Public Health

No more dynamic field exists in medicine today than preventive medicine and public health.* The changes in this area have been greater in the last two decades than in other divisions of medicine because of the opportunities that they have offered for applying on a wide scale the benefits of the rapid advances that have taken place in medical and basic scientific knowledge. Medicine is becoming more complex, so that organization of larger units of persons highly trained in medicine, nursing, the social, biologic and physical sciences, as well as less well-trained therapists and technicians, is needed

---

* This chapter has to do with the work of physicians who deal with various organized medical activities that benefit groups of persons as contrasted with that of physicians who work largely in a direct one-to-one relation with individual patients. Many names have been and are applied to this area—public health, preventive medicine, social medicine, administrative medicine, for example, each of which is often used with different meanings by different persons. Arguing about these differences seems to be unimportant. The purpose of the author in this chapter is to give a brief glimpse into a rapidly expanding field in medicine.

to bring the fruits of modern research to the people. The social concepts of our times have also expanded. Modern societies, in underdeveloped countries as well as those that are highly advanced, are demanding the latest and the best in medicine for all the people. People know more about medical affairs and their demands for service are increasing. In our own affluent society more and more people have the means to pay for medical care, so that the economic barriers to securing it are melting away. In fact, in our own country, the large barriers today are the lack of trained personnel, the poor use of existing personnel, the duplication of services— a series of problems associated essentially with better organization and finding new and more efficient ways to bring better medical care to a whole community—problems that are of immediate concern to the public health expert, if this term is used in its widest sense, as it will be in this chapter.

All of these factors, coupled with the greatly increased populations all over the world and the belief that the enjoyment of health is a reasonable aspiration for everyone, have created an unprecedented demand for health services of all kinds. The challenge is to find the ways to supply the desires of so many people. New ways of organizing and delivering medical service and of preventing disease and disability are essential. Little wonder that experienced physicians specializing in this broad field are in such short supply.

The day has passed when the public health physician spends his time tacking up quarantine signs and looking into privies. In the past his major efforts were devoted to the control of communicable diseases, particularly the handicapping, killing disease of infancy and early childhood. This was important, crucial work. One by one, however, as the frontiers of scientific knowledge have been extended, these cripplers and killers—smallpox, typhoid, plague, malaria, yellow fever, diphtheria, hookworm, cholera, dysentery, pneumonia—have been brought under control. Poliomyelitis is yielding.

During this time emphasis was placed on primary prevention whenever possible. Often a wide variety of community personnel and facilities, medical and nonmedical, were needed before the environment could be controlled or changed, so that enough persons were individually protected. The control of these diseases has been responsible for the increasing span of life over the past half century in more developed countries and for the rapidly declining death rates in certain less well-developed ones in the past decade.

Public health work is one of the youngest branches of public service. Though nurtured through its infancy by the physician, the bacteriologist, the sanitary engineer and the social reformer, it is now growing into maturity with the aid of a host of other professionally trained persons—the physical scientist, the publicist, the educator, the biologist, the dentist, the social scientist (anthropologist, sociologist and psychologist), the social worker, the radio and television expert and the expert in business and management. In the intricate scheme of administering various health plans, craftsmen of great variety and of varying degrees of skill are necessary— and the physician is usually the one chosen to head the team; to plan and direct the service.

Fortunately, public health is rich in drama and adventure and has attracted many creative and brilliant minds. Those who work in its ranks find a rich reward in the public service that they render.

Preventive Medicine is not the exclusive domain of public health. The whole evolution of medical science in the past 20 years has been toward preventive medicine. A larger and larger portion of all medical practice is becoming preventive in every sense of the word. Working together, the public health physician and the private practitioner maintain for the people of the nation a high level of health and medical care. The public health physician does not compete with private practice but rather complements it.

Who is the public health physician of today? Where does he work? What are the duties and the responsibilities of the generalist and the specialist in this field? What kind of medicine do they practice? What training is required? What are the rewards?

Some act chiefly as medical administrators. As such they are employed in many health and medical services that deal with individuals, groups or communities. They run health departments, health centers and hospitals. They administer special projects, such as home-care programs in hospitals, research programs and disease control campaigns. They direct prepayment insurance plans, medical care service programs, voluntary health agencies, medical and related education organizations and international health projects.

The modern public health physician is a practitioner of preventive medicine and, as in other specialties, there is a prescribed program of training leading to Board qualification. He often serves as a health officer, administering a large variety of health activities and programs. In his work, he acts as the leader of an interdisciplinary team and has contact with many health and community groups. In distinction from the practicing physician, the whole community is his patient. As a generalist, he directs the public health program of a given local area, such as a county, a city, a multicounty, a state. What he does depends somewhat on the extent of the health program he finds when he takes the job but very largely too on his own skill and imagination in developing the services needed to meet the community's needs.

To help him administer the health program the health officer works with various physicians who are specialists in their own fields. For instance, the physician in charge of child health is usually a pediatrician as well as a public health specialist. The epidemiologist is a specialist in those forms of medical investigation varying from communicable to chronic diseases. Other specialists include the orthopedist, the virologist, the laboratory director, the internist, the medical care and hospital administrator. The health officer also utilizes the technical skills of cardiologists, psychologists, medical social workers, nutritionists, economists, educators, sociologists. His work involves active co-operation with hos-

208 *Leona Baumgartner and Robert E. Rothermel*

pitals, practicing physicians, housing officials, educational and recreational groups, industrial and labor organizations.

The physician in public health must see the health problems of the community as well as those of the individual. He must see health and disease in their biologic and social relations. The public health physician has the community for his patient, and the community is as varied and complex as the human body.

The health officer, the generalist, needs to know the history of his community, its type of government and record of disease, its present morbidity and mortality picture, environmental sanitation, housing, recreation facilities, hospital and educational facilities, research potentialities, sewage disposal, water supply and its treatment, public attitude toward personal health and the health of the community. He must know the kind of people with whom he will work, their racial origin and how they live.

The specialist in public health, whether he be concerned with maternal and child health programs, cancer or rheumatic fever control, the administration of hospitals, medical care programs or insurance schemes, will also want to know more than his immediate specialty. He will need to look at the many forces that are related to success or failure in meeting the particular goals of his particular program.

As a medical specialist in public health he directs important programs of disease control such as those for the eradication of venereal disease, tuberculosis, rheumatic fever and other communicable diseases. He initiates and directs programs for early diagnosis of cervical cancer, early casefinding of diabetes and glaucoma, the control of radiation, as well as programs designed to uncover new technics in disease prevention and casefinding for early and more conclusive diagnosis. He may be working to improve rehabilitation facilities or centers for cardiac surgery. He conducts research into such new and challenging areas as the relation of diet to heart disease or of smoking to lung cancer or the problems of rehabilitation, economics, narcotic control, alcoholism, environmental pollution, chronic and degenerative diseases and mental health. He is studying home, traffic and occupational accidents—one of today's leading causes of disability and death—and the methods of their prevention. He often has direct connections with a large laboratory service.

Today's public health physician must be research-minded. Research lies at the very root of the performance of good public health practice. Somewhat neglected for three decades, research has in the past decade come to the fore. The problems presented are endless and demand the co-operation of many research disciplines.

Thus, the opportunities for physicians to practice in the field of public health vary widely. They extend to the four corners of the earth and even in this atomic age into outer space. The public health physician has the world as his field of endeavor. Public health specialists are now facing the unprecedented and gigantic problem of world health, sharing with the underdeveloped countries the accumulated experience of the western world in combating the ills of mankind.

Western experience is saving not just decades but centuries for countries abroad. Underdeveloped countries do not have to rediscover smallpox vaccine or penicillin. But even these standard operating procedures and their application cannot simply be transplanted *in toto* into a strange and different environment. It requires a dynamic and perceptive public health worker to adapt this western technology to the native environment. The skills of the anthropologist, the political scientist, the economist are called upon. These world health workers make unique and original contributions to the substance of medicine and the technology of public health.

A large share of the international health program is carried on through the World Health Organization, though there are also opportunities to work with other governmental and industrial groups. The activities include highly specialized programs related to malaria, tuberculosis, venereal diseases and sanitation. They include the important functions of examining the public health administration, professional education and health education requirements of the countries involved.

There are two aspects to international public health activities in the underdeveloped countries. One is the technical aspect; it is fairly easy. However, the other, the nontechnical aspect, presents many new and challenging problems. How are we to get the procedures, the technology we know about, accepted and incorporated into the routines and the life values of these countries? How to persuade the population to accept, support and co-operate is the real task for public health administration. This is an area where cultural and sociologic differences are very important. The physicians and the public health personnel who sign up to serve in these campaigns have much first-hand experience in anthropology.

The Commissioned Corps of the United States Public Health Service is an organization that offers many opportunities for public health physicians both at home and abroad. Abroad they serve on medical missions, special details for study and consultation, on assignment to consulates and embassies. At home they have the satisfaction of serving in a vigorous professional organization that is assisting states and communities in developing a modern nationwide health program. Opportunities for advancement are afforded in three fields: clinical medicine, research and public health. Training is available to the physician either for certification by a recognized specialty board or for intensive training in public health, clinical practice or administration. Service in the Commissioned Corps offers the physician an interesting and challenging career in public health and administrative medicine, with opportunity for steady advancement and security when he retires.

Training for Public Health and Certification in the Specialty. Physicians entering the field of public health require specialized training, in addition to a working knowledge of a wide range of medical subjects. Because the scope of the health officer's work goes beyond the field of medicine, he requires some knowledge of engineering, environmental sanitation, health education, behavioral sciences, community leadership, political science and the laboratory sciences as related to public health. He learns the technics of epidemiology and biostatistics, as well as understanding the social organization and the structure of his particular community. He needs to learn or to know how to get along with people. The basic sciences of public health—biometrics, epidemiology, community organization and public health administration—bear the same relation to the practice of public health as do the basic sciences to the practice of medicine.

As with the private physician, the public health physician never stands still. Medical science is an especially rapid marcher, and the social sciences are progressing rapidly in the present day. The public health worker who fails to keep up with the advances in related sciences, who does not grow with or faster than the job, soon becomes a handicap to himself and his organization.

The medical graduate becomes a specialist in public health through specialized training and experience. Training for the generalist, at least, is best done in an accredited residency training area. These are in 18 states, which, with the numerous local areas within them are listed in the Annual Internship and Residency Number of the *Journal of the American Medical Association.*

Training includes one year at a recognized school of public health leading to the degree of Master of Public Health. There are 13 schools of public health* located in the United States and Canada. Stipends to residents range from about $5,000 to $9,500 for field training. Stipends and tuition are also paid during the academic year.

It should be emphasized that there are many opportunities for physicians to work in public health without such extended training. The certified pediatrician, internist or orthopedist, for example, with an interest other than the care of his individual patients will find opportunities to assist in or direct

---

* California, Columbia, Harvard, Johns Hopkins, Michigan, Minnesota, Montreal, North Carolina, Pittsburgh, Puerto Rico, Toronto, Tulane, Yale.

community activities related to his specialty through government agencies, the voluntary health agencies, labor groups,
and so forth. He will usually find that some courses outside
his specialty will help him on the new job.

The American Board of Preventive Medicine was established as a Specialty Board in 1949. To be eligible to take
the examinations a physician must have completed two years
of supervised training in an accredited residency, one year of
academic study at a school of public health for the M.P.H.
degree, and three additional years of responsible full-time
experience in public health or a related field.

There are now about 2000 Board-certified public health
specialists in the United States, dedicated to their tasks and
respected by their colleagues in private practice. There are
more than 1000 members of the American College of Preventive Medicine, all recognized by the American Medical
Association. Public health is represented by a big and rapidly
growing medical specialist group.

Salaries vary widely, but physicians in public health have
the advantages of a good, stable income, enhanced by the fact
that there is no capital investment required for an office or
equipment or office personnel. Hours are reasonable and relatively stable, with practically none of the irregular demands
of private practice. Other benefits are opportunities for promotion, insurance plans, vacation and sick leave allowances
and good retirement plans. Joint appointments on medical
school faculties are often available for those well enough
qualified.

Full-time positions are not difficult to obtain, although as
in any other profession the beginner is not always able to work
exactly where he desires to be. Building a good reputation,
scholastically and in one's first job, makes moving to the more
desired position relatively simple, since the demand for
trained and experienced physicians in this field is now so
large.

To determine the available opportunities for a career in
public health or administrative medicine, one should check

with his city, county or state health department; with hospitals; with other official and voluntary medical and health agencies on the city, state or federal levels. The American Public Health Association, 1790 Broadway, New York 19, N. Y., serves as a clearing-house for job openings in all areas of public health.

The medical student interested in public health can often find summer scholarships for work of various kinds. There are also attractive training jobs available for the graduate at the Communicable Disease Center in Atlanta.

The Future of Public Health. What are the futures in this broad field? For many reasons they seem to be boundless. New discoveries in the physical and chemical sciences and an expanding technology continue to create new hazards for mankind. In fact, the chief deterrents to health in the future appear to be manmade. The effects of ionizing radiation and food additives are only two examples recently recognized. Further developments in medical genetics may well lead to greater understanding of the pathogenesis of many diseases, particularly the metabolic disorders. These may require new environmental controls. But even within the confines of existing knowledge there is much yet to be done in controlling or ameliorating the effects of the chronic diseases—diabetes, heart disease, arthritis, cerebral accidents, cancer, glaucoma. Mental illness, alcoholism, narcotic addiction, air pollution and rehabilitation of many kinds present new challenges.

Successful attacks on the problems call for skills and knowledge similar to those that led to the conquest of the communicable disease. The future belongs to those who will create it.

W. BARRY WOOD, JR., M.D.

Professor of Microbiology at Johns Hopkins University

20

The Medical Sciences

The most important single advance in medicine since the turn of the century has not been a specific discovery that has revolutionized clinical practice, such as that of insulin, or of penicillin; rather it has been the fact that physicians in general have been forced by the pressures of progress to become better scientists. Instead of being trained as artisans in a trade, in which dogma was often passed down uncritically from generation to generation, modern doctors have been educated as university graduate students. Taught by men actively engaged in the pursuit of new knowledge, they have been brought up both to expect and to accept discoveries that will compel them to alter their methods of practice. In fact, they quickly learn that the greatest challenge of their professional careers is that of keeping well enough abreast of scientific progress to bring to their patients the best that medicine has to offer.

This endless task has become particularly difficult of late, primarily because of a striking change that has taken place in the nature of medical research. Whereas the advances of medicine only a generation or two ago were essentially descriptive and were made for the most part by alert physicians working at the bedside, they come today from basic science and clinical research laboratories where the newest and most sophisticated technics of chemistry, physics and biology are applied to essentially mechanistic studies of disease. For only from knowledge of the deranged mechanisms of illness do optimal methods of treatment eventually emerge. Also, like modern biology, modern medicine has "gone molecular." Comprehension of disease mechanisms in the gross, as it were, is no longer sufficient; they must be understood at the molecular level. This means more biochemistry and more biophysics in every branch of medicine. To remain effective throughout their professional careers, doctors must now possess a deeper and broader knowledge of the preclinical sciences than ever before.

How are they to master and keep up with these rapidly expanding subjects? Surely they can do so only if they are exposed to sound preclinical teaching in medical school, and only if they remain, in fact, alert students of medical science for the rest of their professional lives. The first of these requirements calls for a further strengthening of the preclinical departments of medical schools; the second bespeaks the need for better methods of continuing education for practicing physicians and surgeons, particularly in the basic sciences.

Fortunately, movements are already afoot that give promise of meeting both of these needs. It was not so many years ago that one of the leading medical schools of the nation was said, by a wise professor from a rival university, to resemble a grand piano with precarious underpinnings of relatively spindly and neglected basic science departments. Such imbalance of clinical and preclinical strengths has been all too common in medical faculties of the past. But measures to correct it have recently been instituted in many universities. Indeed, the increasing importance of basic science in modern medicine has made such corrective changes inevitable. So, too, has the rapidly expanding volume of medical research. A rough idea of the recent growth of the latter may be gained from examining the Federal appropriations for the National Institutes of Health, which provides a major share of the financial support for the nation's medical research. In 1947 its research budget was $8.4 million; by 1960 the same budget had risen to $283.8 million, more than $200 million of which was assigned to projects and training programs in universities and teaching hospitals, exclusive of the National Institutes of Health. The funneling of a large proportion of this money into the medical schools has had a profound effect upon their development. New buildings have been erected, new laboratories opened, and new faculty positions created. The resulting additions in facilities and staff have not only improved laboratories for clinical research but also have revitalized basic science departments. In fact, in many instances they have gone a long way toward correcting the imbalance between preclinical and clinical resources.

Nor is the need for more basic science appreciated only by university faculties; the demand of practicing physicians for postgraduate instruction in preclinical subjects has also risen sharply. To cite but a single example, the American College of Physicians, which is the national society for practitioners of internal medicine, sponsors each year a scientific meeting designed to provide postgraduate instruction for its large membership. Until very recently, all but a handful of the papers presented were "purely clinical." In 1960, however, a major section of the program was devoted to "Basic Medical Science Sessions." Here are the titles of some of the papers:

> Structure-Function Relationships in Viruses
> Genetics of Viruses
> Antibiotics as Inhibitors of Bacterial Wall Synthesis
> The Present Status of Starling's Law of the Heart
> Regulation of Blood and Fluid Volume in the Lung
> Gene Structure and Gene Function
> Medical Applications of Human Cell Cultures
> Current Status of Neuropharmacology
> Lipogenesis and Cholesterologenesis
> Fat Mobilization and Transport
> Viruses and Cancer
> Relation of Cyclic Adenylic Acid to Hormone Action

These subjects were not imposed upon the audience as propaganda from "the ivory tower"; they were advisedly selected by the society's own program committee. Their nature clearly indicates that the informed membership of the American College of Physicians is keenly aware of the importance of postgraduate instruction in the most basic aspects of pre-clinical science.

But what do these trends have to do with the choice of a career in medicine? Obviously a great deal, for they are the indicators of the future character of medicine as a profession. They are signposts which everyone contemplating a medical career should examine with the greatest of care.

I have recently heard two college presidents make the same statement about premedical students: namely, that they constitute the most highly motivated group in the student body. That this is so in many colleges I have little doubt, because premedical students have before them a very definite goal. To attain it, they know that they must do better than average work at college. With all of the medical schools of the country able to accept only about half of those who apply, the competition for admission is exceptionally stiff. Of these "facts of life" all premedical students are fully cognizant. What is not so clear to them is the wide variety of careers that will be open to them if they make the grade.

Nine times out of ten a person interested in medicine has as his sole objective a career in clinical practice. This is exactly as it should be, since the primary mission of the profession is to treat and prevent illness. And surely there are few more gratifying callings in society than that of being a good doctor. He is "one of the most advanced types of human being on earth today," wrote the philosopher Whitehead, in 1941. "He is skeptical toward the data of his own profession, welcomes discoveries which upset his previous hypotheses, and is still animated by human sympathy and understanding."

But the changing trends in medicine, to which I have referred, are creating new patterns of professional opportunities for medical graduates. Although clinical practice still claims by far the greatest number of M.D.'s, there is now an increasing demand for physician-research scientists, physician-administrators and physician-teachers. The need for physician-research scientists has, of course, been created by the growing volume of medical research. The need for physician-administrators stems not only from developments in public health (to which Dr. Baumgartner has alluded in the preceding chapter), but also to the increasingly complex operations of hospitals, medical schools, and fund-granting agencies supporting medical education and research. And the need for more physician-teachers results from enlargement of existing medical schools, the creation of new ones and the ever-increasing demand for more postgraduate education.

Thus the medical graduate of today may become a practicing physician, a research-scientist, a medical administrator or a teacher. What happens, in fact, is that many doctors, particularly in university communities, follow combined careers. It is traditional, for example, in most university hospitals, for the clinical staff to engage in both practice and teaching, or in teaching and clinical research, or even in all three. Likewise, in the preclinical departments of medical schools, the faculty is usually occupied with research as well as with teaching. In nonuniversity communities, on the other hand, clinical practice alone, or full-time administration in a health department or other agency is the rule.

How does one choose between these alternatives? And when must the decision be made? Specific answers obviously cannot be given to either of these questions, but two pertinent generalities are worth bearing in mind.

First, it should be understood from the outset that no one of the alternative careers in medicine is necessarily any *better* than another. Though they differ in character, they are all of essentially equal importance. Indeed, society can enjoy the full benefits of modern medicine only if practice, research, administration and teaching are all performed by dedicated and competent individuals. Second, all require the best possible kind of medical education. Therefore, students entering medical school need not waste their time worrying about what they are going to do after graduation; rather, they should devote their entire energies to learning as much medical science as possible during their four years as medical undergraduates.

Of every class that is graduated from medical school, all but a few will elect to become hospital interns and later, residents. Most of these will go directly into clinical practice, once they have completed their hospital training. Some will take graduate fellowships in either clinical or preclinical departments to prepare themselves for the practice of one or another specialty. Of those who take specialty training a few will remain in university faculties, as teachers and clinical investigators; the rest will become the practicing specialists of their communities. A small number of those who complete hospital house-officerships will ultimately become health officers or medical administrators.

In every graduating class, however, there will also be a few students who will wish to enter full-time careers in academic medicine. Unlike the majority, whose greatest satisfactions will be derived from the personal relations involved in helping and caring for sick patients as individuals, this small group will be attracted to teaching and research by a desire to have the time and the opportunity to work at the frontiers of knowledge and to share with students the thrills of learning and discovery. For these few, the challenges of study and research will outweigh the more direct and tangible satisfactions of serving the sick.

Why should anyone be so attracted to scientific research? Innate curiosity is probably the most important motivating force of all. I can still remember how I was first made aware of its significance. While an undergraduate in college, I had the privilege of working in the laboratory of the distinguished scientist and philosopher, Lawrence J. Henderson, known to most biochemistry students as the co-author of the Henderson-Hasselbach equation. One day, when I was indulging in some starry-eyed speculations as to possible applications of the work I was doing, he brought me abruptly to earth by saying, "For one engaged in scientific research, a desire to benefit

mankind is a poor substitute for curiosity." My first reaction
was one of disillusionment. As a prospective medical student
my primary purpose in life was "to benefit mankind." What
did he really mean? It was not until some time later, when I
had gained a little more experience in the laboratory, that
I began to appreciate the point he was trying to impress upon
me, namely, that to do significant research, one must be
genuinely interested in solving a problem for its own sake.
Only an abiding curiosity in the answer *per se* will generate
the kind of patience and tenacity needed for ultimate success.

For those who aspire to full-time careers in medical science,
three types of opportunities are available. Each has its special
appeal. First, there are jobs in both industrial and non-indus-
trial research institutes, where staff members have essentially
no teaching responsibilities and, therefore, can devote practically all of their time to research. Such positions naturally
do not long satisfy those who have an urge to work with students. Secondly, there are clinical research opportunities in
university hospitals and medical schools, where it is possible
for one to engage in scientific investigations having a direct
bearing upon clinical medicine. To many this is an ideal
kind of university appointment, because it combines not only
teaching and research, but it also brings the worker into intimate contact with the fascinating problems of disease. And
lastly, there are faculty positions in medical school departments of anatomy, physiology, biochemistry, biophysics, pharmacology, microbiology and pathology. What are the particular attractions of full-time careers in these preclinical
departments? To this question I can only speak for myself. To
me there appear to be two.

The most important one has to do with the relation of the
preclinical sciences to medicine in particular and to the rest
of natural science in general. In contrast with clinical medicine, the preclinical disciplines have to do almost entirely
with principles that have no direct bearing on the practi-
calities of patient care. And yet, as I have already stressed, it
is upon these basic principles that the advances of clinical

practice are eventually built. In other words, the preclinical scientist works at the foundations of medicine, between the clinicians, on the one hand, and the biologists, the physicists and the chemists, on the other. Here he studies, in an enviable environment, where the opportunities to probe the phenomena of human biology are unexcelled.

The second attraction has to do with a very practical matter, namely that of *time*. In regard to this priceless commodity, preclinical scientists have a definite advantage over most other medical graduates, for, unlike their clinical colleagues, they carry none of the time-consuming responsibilities of patient care—responsibilities which, no matter how limited, must have the top priority in the life of anyone who is worthy of assuming them. This fact alone gives the preclinical scientist significantly more time for research and study.

Finally, I should like to add a word about preparation for careers in preclinical science. In the preceding discussion, I have referred almost exclusively to doctors of medicine. However, all preclinical teachers and investigators are not, and certainly need not be, medical graduates. On the contrary, the over-all strength of a preclinical department depends upon a liberal scattering of Ph.D.'s whose depth of knowledge in one or another of the natural sciences is greater than that of most medical doctors. Indeed, many of the most distinguished preclinical departments of the world are headed by men who have never gone to medical school. Conversely, completion of the usual medical curriculum, and even clinical experience as a hospital intern and resident, may serve as excellent preparation for a preclinical career. Possessed of a first-hand knowledge of medicine, and thus aware of the special problems that confront medical students, individuals with such a background often develop into outstanding teachers. There is obviously no ideal course that everyone should follow. The one essential prerequisite is a sound training in basic science.

The kind of scientific experience needed is not provided by the standard medical curriculum; it must be supplemented by a number of years of study and research in a basic science department. In order to allow medical students to get a start in such extracurricular work, many medical schools in recent years have developed extensive student-research programs. The majority have involved summer fellowships, but some have also utilized blocks of free time made available during the academic year. At Johns Hopkins University, for example, a newly designed curriculum affords special opportunities for students desiring research experience during the course of their regular medical education. It not only includes free time, in solid blocks of ten weeks, during each of the last three years of medical school, but it also permits properly qualified college students to begin their medical studies a year earlier than usual. The year thus gained in time may then be utilized for special studies, including research fellowships. In addition, a provision has been made for students who drop out for a year's special work, to accelerate their required clinical courses in the last two years and thus graduate with their own classes. Both of the last two features, which are made possible by slightly extended academic years, allow students to spend as much as twelve consecutive months in full-time research, without requiring an extra year.

Innovations of this sort, which are taking different forms in different universities, afford new opportunities for training in research. One of their principal objectives is to increase the man-power pool of teachers and investigators, who are well enough grounded in the preclinical disciplines to assure the continued advance of medical science.

ROBERT E. STOWELL, M.D., PH.D.

Scientific Director, Armed Forces Institute of Pathology

21

Pathology

Pathology is the science of the study of the causes, the processes and the effects of disease. As a practitioner of a medical
specialty, the pathologist is a doctor's doctor applying laboratory medicine to the problem of the patient. As a basic scientist, he utilizes the technics and the knowledge of anatomy,
physiology, biochemistry, microbiology and biophysics. In
many situations the pathologist is the expert to whom the
clinician turns for the great assistance that laboratory medicine is contributing increasingly to modern patient care.
Because of the many fields in which the pathologist is often
expected to be competent, he has been considered by some as
a scientific generalist, in contrast with the scientific specialist
who strives to learn more and more information about fewer
and narrower subjects.

The pathologist's activities are not restricted to one field.
The scope of pathology is as great as the diversity of life; all
forms of life are potentially subject to disease. Hence, the
discipline of pathology is restricted only by the scientific curiosity, the imagination and the competence of the individual.

Few people have any idea of the nature of the pathologist's
day-to-day work or the central role he plays in the practice of
modern scientific medicine. Most patients do not understand
that the decision as to whether they will be treated for cancer,
syphilis or amebiasis may depend more on the skills of the
pathologist than on those of the private physician. The patient

does not know to what an extent his health and even his life depend on the precision and the judgment with which laboratory tests are carried out and interpreted.

Pathology, one of the most important disciplines of modern medicine, had its scientific origin in the Middle Ages. The early contributions to pathology were made by medical practitioners, and it was not until the 19th century that some physicians began to devote their full time to the specialty. Excellent reviews of training[1] and of the history of pathology[2] are available.

Many other clinical and basic science specialists beside those who devote their full time to the discipline make some important contributions to pathology. About 3 per cent of the certified medical specialists are qualified pathologists. Pathology is one of the most rapidly developing fields from the standpoint of new knowledge, technics and the number of specialists in the field; yet twice as many of these specialists could be used as are presently available.

CHALLENGES OF THE STUDY OF DISEASE

In terms of significance to society, to biologic and medical sciences and to the individual scientist, pathology presents some of the most stimulating opportunities and challenges within the broad area of scientific endeavor. Most pathologists are concerned in varying degrees with consultation, research, education and administration.

Service to Society and Medicine. Laboratory medicine shares with other clinical disciplines in contributing great benefits to society through better patient care. In addition, pathologists through their research often make very great contributions to new scientific knowledge capable of serving mankind. The pathologist is a very important member of the modern team of research scientists contributing to the advancement of medical sciences through investigation and teaching.

Personal Satisfactions. How should a medical student select a field for medical specialization? First, each must be aware of his own interests, personality traits, emotional and intellectual needs, goals and capabilities, and then evaluate these in the light of the opportunities in various specialties of potential interest to him.

All types of medical practice are important to human welfare, but by reason of temperament, interest or aptitude not all physicians are equally suited to become pathologists. Specialization in pathology will be most gratifying to one who in the practice of medicine prefers to use relatively precise laboratory methods and to be a consultant to the physician directly responsible for the patient's care.

Interest tests by psychologists have shown that pathologists prefer to work with factual data rather than with abstract ideas. The interests of pathologists are more like those of chemists than those of other specialists. Pathologists have more interests in common with internists than they do with surgeons.

The substantial professional satisfaction that the pathologist finds in his daily work is of prime importance. No matter how great a role the pathologist may play in preventing a needless operation or even saving a patient's life, his part in advising and guiding the personal physician in the care and the treatment of the patient tends to be cloaked in anonymity so far as the patient is concerned. Personal satisfaction must come rather from deep inner knowledge that his important aid reaches many more patients, as well as their physicians, than he could serve as a personal physician at their bedside.

If self-fulfillment dictates that the young doctor have a close physician-patient relationship, then pathology is not the career for him. If, on the other hand, he can obtain deep inner satisfaction from the laboratory rather than from the sick patient, from dealing with other physicians rather than with patients, from broad rather than limited pursuits in medicine and from a scientific life of contemplation, investigation and analysis—then he might well consider pathology for his career.

Although pathologists may not receive acclaim from patients, they are among those specialists who hold the highest regard of medical students and professional colleagues. Six pathologists have received international recognition in the form of Nobel Prizes for their research contributions.

The pathologist is free from many of the concerns of his clinical colleagues. He is relatively free of unpredictable demands on his professional time. He has few night calls or interrupted meals, and he may enjoy time for his family, community activities and even a vacation! These factors may account for a greater life expectancy than that of many other specialists.

In hospitals an established practice awaits the pathologist's demonstration of his skills. The better he serves his colleagues and their patients, the more his assistance will be requested. In general, each new therapeutic agent and laboratory instrument creates more work for the pathologist; future unemployment is inconceivable for the competent. Increasing demands of our country for medical care, research and educational facilities all provide increasing needs and opportunities for pathologists.

Tools to practice precise laboratory medicine are at hand, and there is less cause for worry over incorrect or presumptive diagnoses or therapy. The institution in which a pathologist works may take care of many of his administrative problems, and so he has more time to devote to scientific matters.

The pathologist deals with medical colleagues on a basis of mutual scientific understanding rather than with patients and their personal complaints. His private life can be lived according to his own sense of values, with freedom from concern about what patients may think. The pathologist's success depends more on his professional competence and integrity than on his social contacts.

A career in pathology offers special attractions for women. To interrupt a professional career in pathology for a year or more and then return to it is easier than in most other specialties. Part-time opportunities, with freedom to attend to family responsibilities, are often available. When their husbands are transferred to another place, married women pathologists find it easier to move because they need not slowly build up a practice in a new location.

By material criteria pathology is among those specialties which are remunerated the best. Because of the shortage of pathologists, incomes tend to start at a good level upon completion of formal training. However, as in all fields of endeavor, one must look beyond monetary considerations, realizing that what income remains after providing for the necessities of life furnishes only such satisfactions as money will buy.

Consultation. Most pathologists devote the major share of their time to medical practice as consultants in laboratory medicine and as advisers to their clinical medical colleagues. What is the clinical significance of the results of a laboratory test for a particular patient? Will this patient's tumor probably respond to x-ray therapy? What were the results of the therapy given the patient? Did the death of the patient result from accidental trauma, for which the relatives hope to collect remuneration, or was death from unrelated causes? In answering such questions, the well-trained pathologist may find himself the busiest consultant on the hospital staff. Although the laboratory is his workshop, as a consultant he may be called to the operating room, to the patient's bedside, or to see the patient as a hematologist. Most pathologists find their consultative practice of medicine a most gratifying and stimulating experience.

Research. Through his diverse investigations the pathologist adds to medical knowledge of the causes, the mechanisms of development and the effects of treatment of disease. Although such research may be highly specialized or basic, one of the great advantages in the approach of the pathologist to research is his breadth of knowledge of basic sciences and methods applicable to the study of human disease. He can be a research generalist or a specialist. The facilities he uses to practice laboratory medicine provide excellent tools for his research.

However, some pathologists use special facilities or technics in their research. The idea that originates with microscopic observations of diseased tissues or unexplained results of a clinical laboratory test sparks the pathologist's creative imagination to apply a variety of modern tools and technics. For example, he may use the electron microscope to study ultrastructural changes in cells, histochemistry to explain altered cellular metabolism, germ-free animals to study antibody reactions or gas chromatography to isolate a new metabolite from the serum. The pathologist has an unusually favorable opportunity for conducting investigations. His horizons need be limited only by his ingenuity, knowledge, needs for special facilities and time to devote to research. A relatively small but increasing number of young, well-trained pathologists are seeking readily available opportunities in which they can devote the major part or all of their efforts to medical research. Such men get their personal satisfaction from the significance of their accomplishment as well as from the knowledge that their research may ultimately benefit thousands of patients rather than just the individual patient whom the private physician serves.

Education. To a greater extent than other medical personnel, most pathologists devote varying amounts of their attention to teaching medical and other colleagues; residents; interns; medical, dental or university students; or paramedical personnel such as technicians, physical therapists or nurses. Because of the authoritative position the pathologist holds as an expert student of disease, there are many opportunities to teach. This important responsibility of communicating knowledge to professional personnel and the general public is a most stimulating and gratifying experience.

The pathologist is an enthusiastic participant at many hospital staff teaching conferences. His up-to-date knowledge of basic sciences is exchanged with clinicians, who in turn keep him abreast of their patients' problems and of new developments in clinical medicine. Many pathologists are in charge of their own medical technology training program and also assist in teaching student nurses and other medical assistants.

Administration. Pathologists have the responsibilities of leadership for the supporting staff who assist them in their practice, in teaching and in research. Because of their broad background and experience, they are often asked to participate on many committees and in administrative functions of the institutes with which they are associated.

In the growth of modern medicine, the hypertrophy of administrative functions and the hyperplasia of committee responsibilities represent a potential hypoplasia of the pathologist's effective scientific pursuits. Some pathologists have become full-time administrators, and a few have become recluses by attempting to close their doors to the demands of administration; most still seek more efficient mechanisms to give vital administrative service with suitable conservation of time and effort.

Interrelationships of These Opportunities. Most pathologists, then, obtain their deep personal satisfaction from a busy professional life involving varying responsibilities in consultation, research, education and administration. Students or practitioners of medicine have little idea of the life of a pathologist unless they spend some time working with one. Fortunately, more students are taking advantage of opportunities to work in the pathologist's laboratory, an experience which so fires their enthusiasm that increasing numbers of better students are deciding to become pathologists. On-the-job experience will continue to be the most effective recruiting mechanism for pathologists. It is best if physicians can have experience in clinical and laboratory medicine before reaching a decision on their careers. Some with aptitude for pathology have been convinced by a clinical internship or externship that they should become pathologists.

Pathology is the most general of medical specialties, since it is concerned with all the other disciplines and specialties that make up medical knowledge. A pathologist should be able to say, "Nothing that pertains to disease is without interest to me."

Most pathologists have at hand the technics of all the basic medical sciences and available laboratory facilities and methods for studies in histology, physiology, hematology, serology, bacteriology and biochemistry. The pathologist has ready access to hospital patients and the operating rooms. As a scientist-consultant and student of disease, he has the opportunity to maintain and perfect his skill as a clinical diagnostician. The results of all laboratory tests, as well as every piece of tissue removed by the surgeon, come to him for his skillful interpretation. He is the physician among all specialists who is regularly afforded the privilege of examining the bodies of deceased patients to study firsthand the outcome of the combat between disease processes and their therapy. He is especially trained in gross and microscopic changes of disease and has available laboratory facilities and technicians to assist him. There are also facilities for laboratory animals for the study of biologic processes of disease.

The specialty is not limited to any one organ, system, or group of diseases, or to one instrument or technic. It is as broad as the field of medicine itself. It provides daily contact with clinical problems of most clinical specialties and offers all the tools and the methods of diverse medical sciences for their solution. It is the court of last resort for the best clinicians in the practical diagnosis and the care of the sick. It is a specialty so centered among other specialties as to provide one man with the best materials and methods of modern medicine for the study of disease.

TRAINING

Most pathologists should obtain adequately broad training to meet future consultative, investigative, educational and administrative responsibilities. The purpose of the first 4 to 7 years of formal postdoctoral training is to prepare the pathologist for more than 40 years of continuing educational experience. Hence, learning suitable concepts and principles is more important than attempting to cram the calvarium with facts, figures and fantasies. Training programs should not become stereotyped to meet prescribed artificial standards; rather, they should be varied within a reasonable range according to the available opportunities, interests of the trainee and his ultimate objectives.

Internships, Residencies and Fellowships. For most, the first year after medical school will be profitably spent in a good mixed or rotating clinical internship. This increases the future pathologist's understanding of clinical medicine and of the way in which pathology can best be applied to its problems. A minimum of 2 years of experience in clinical pathology and 2 years in anatomic pathology are recommended for general training. Training in both clinical and anatomic pathology provides a much better background for general pathology than more specialized training and at the same time is an excellent basis on which to superimpose more specialized experience.

Fortunately, there is considerable flexibility in some training programs, and a wide choice of programs is available in many different institutions. By a small percentage of trainees in pathology, consideration should be given to other types of training. A few can acquire knowledge in 2 years that would take most people 4 years and an occasional person 6 years. Some may want to train primarily in anatomic pathology, and others chiefly in clinical pathology; those who want to do research only will be helped by some general training in pathology. Under special circumstances, such as specialized interests or pressure of training time, a straight internship in pathology in lieu of a clinical internship has merit. It is of little consequence whether the trainee is called a resident or a fellow.

How does a young doctor choose a place to train in pathology? He should attempt to define his goals and then seek the best opportunities to meet these objectives. He should talk with the directors of several different types of pathology programs, and he should talk especially with the current trainees regarding their experiences. He should consider first training with a pathologist who is doing the type and the caliber of work that he himself would most like to do someday.

Graduate Degree. A few pathologists, as a part of their formal training, obtain a graduate degree, such as a master of science or a doctor of philosophy in pathology or in other basic science subjects. This experience may be excellent training for research; equally good experience can be obtained in less formal programs in some other medical centers. In general, the caliber of graduate programs and medical-center fellowships established for research pathologists in recent years is good. However, the mark of a scientist should be his competence and accomplishments rather than the number of degrees listed after his name. The young doctor who wishes to become a pathologist should seek a formal graduate program only if it provides the training he wants, and not because of anticipated prestige.

American Board of Pathology. This specialty Board has established minimum standards for training and certification in diagnostic pathology. Of the 4,000 Board pathologists living in August, 1962, 50 per cent were certified in anatomic pathology; 5 per cent, in clinical pathology; and 45 per cent, in anatomic and clinical pathology. Five per cent of certified pathologists also held a certificate in one of the special fields of forensic pathology, neuropathology, clinical microbiology, clinical chemistry and hematology. The Board recognizes a wide variety of types of training programs.[3]

GENERAL CAREER OPPORTUNITIES

According to their interests and goals, pathologists enjoy one of the greatest varieties of choice of career opportunities.

Private Laboratory Practice. A pathologist in such practice performs useful service by aiding many physicians and patients who send or bring material to him for laboratory study from their offices or hospitals. This type of practice provides more independence to one or more pathologists who own the practice, employ personnel and make all necessary arrangements to provide service and collect fees from patients. Some pathologists are also concerned with laboratory cardiology, electrocardiography, radioisotopes, laboratory aspects of annual physical and toxicologic examinations for industry, and insurance programs.

Hospital Practice. The largest number of pathologists carry out their practice in a hospital, in which are found excellent opportunities for service to patients, teaching and often research. If all the available facilities and opportunities of an ordinary hospital were inventoried and then a plan prepared which would be designed to give one staff member the best of everything available for the comprehensive study of disease, the result would be very close to the opportunities that most hospital pathologists enjoy every day. In small hospitals the pathologist is one of the most readily available physicians, and he frequently consults with staff and hospital administrators on many matters and supervises training and research programs.

Sometimes a pathologist will serve more than one hospital or will accept specimens sent to him from outside the institution. Usually the hospital provides the pathologist with certain laboratory facilities and administrative assistance, and the pathologist supervises laboratory personnel and bills patients for his services. On the basis of a negotiated contract, the pathologist may be guaranteed a minimum income and pay a percentage of receipts to the hospital for the facilities provided.

Each hospital of over 100 or 200 beds should have a pathologist; many institutions do not have sufficient pathology service available. Increasingly, two or more pathologists are organizing a group practice to serve one or more laboratories or hospitals. This type of organization has certain advantages in terms of service to patients, consultation and sharing the work, vacation, research and educational opportunities.

Research Institutes. Most medical research institutes already have or are presently seeking pathologists for their staffs. Because of the shortage of well-trained pathologists, some pharmaceutical firms and research institutes have of necessity employed veterinary pathologists or biologists who were relatively untrained in pathology. The research institutes usually provide excellent research facilities but little opportunity for teaching or diagnostic human pathology within the institute. The salaries vary considerably but are about the same as those for many universities.

Medical Schools. Many medical schools provide the best opportunities for pathologists who want a stimulating teaching environment, good research facilities and consultation on well-documented patient problems. Many departments of pathology have been improved and strengthened in recent years, with increased geographic full-time staffs and new or renovated buildings. In some instances subspecialties of pathology have been brought together, with consequent improvement of teaching and training. The importance of improved training in clinical pathology has been recognized increasingly. The advent of ample monies for research has increased staff requirements, and many departments have one or more vacancies.

Many young pathologists spend several highly productive years in a university medical center before they leave salaried positions for more remunerative practice. The medical school professor, although he is in the top percentiles of income for our country, receives more of his compensation in personal gratification and less in the coin of the realm than his colleagues in the hospital or in private practice. Many other pathologists participate part time in teaching or research at medical schools.

Government Service. Pathologists in government service constitute a large group under municipal, state or federal administration. They are employed in a large variety of institutions, including general or special hospitals, medical schools and research or other kinds of institutes. Opportunities cover a broad spectrum that does not facilitate generalizations, especially in municipal and state institutions.

Federal Institutions. The Public Health Service, the Navy, the Air Force, the Army and the Department of Defense maintain one or more outstanding institutes each, with superb facilities for practicing pathology, research and postdoctoral education. In addition to their commissioned officers, both the Armed Forces Institute of Pathology and the National Institutes of Health employ a number of civil service pathologists. Many of the Veterans Administration hospitals are associated with medical schools and to varying degrees share their benefits. The Veterans Administration, the military services and the Public Health Service each offer career residency programs that provide relatively good stipends and require obligated repayment in the form of years of continued service according to the length of training supported. There are about 640 qualified pathologists and 240 trainees employed full time by the United States Government.

The relatively high standards of work in pathology in many Federal hospitals are aided by consultants, training programs, extramural standards, regulations and liaison with the Armed Forces Institute of Pathology. Since patients are not billed for individual laboratory procedures, there is less concern about carrying out desired scientific tests because of the patient's inability to pay. Remuneration according to regulated pay scales provides relatively good beginning stipends, which increase slowly but provide security, and survivor, retirement and other benefits. For military and Public Health Service officers, there are provisions for the use of the commissary, medical care for officers and dependents, and income tax savings based on exclusion of quarters and rations payments for tax purposes. After 20 or more years of Federal service, many pathologists draw liberal retirement pay while carrying on a full-time practice in civilian medicine. There are regular working hours and opportunities for travel.

SPECIAL CAREER FIELDS

In addition to the broad background of pathology, of which most should have reasonable understanding, many pathologists specialize to a high degree in one or more of the many aspects of the study of disease. Although originally clinicians were their own pathologists, increasingly they have recognized the need for full-time specialists in this field. Even in those few areas in which the clinician-specialists are presently doing much of their work in pathology, such as in ophthalmology, otolaryngology and dermatology, within a decade or two their pathology will probably be done largely by specialist-pathologists. In other basic sciences, such as in chemistry and microbiology, the rapid scientific advances are being met in special circumstances by Ph.D.'s co-operating with pathologists to form laboratory medicine teams in which the pathologist gives leadership and medical guidance.

The many special fields of anatomic pathology comprise all the organ systems, including neuropathology, cardiovascular, gynecologic, endocrine, ophthalmologic, otorhinolaryngologic and dermatologic pathology,[4] as well as surgical pathology and exfoliative cytology. The principal subspecialties of clinical pathology include hematology, clinical chemistry, microbiology, serology and blood banking. Other special fields that are neither primarily anatomic nor clinical pathology include immunopathology, radiopathology, forensic, pediatric, geriatric, geographic, experimental and comparative pathology.

FUTURE OPPORTUNITIES

In the past century, following Virchow's initiation of the study of disease at the cellular level, pathology has witnessed continually advancing horizons. In the past decade studies have been undertaken by pathologists and others at the ultrastructural level with the electron microscope. The next decade will see increasing emphasis on molecular pathology[5] to explain disease. New technology, including automation and electronic data processing, will move into the pathologist's laboratory to increase greatly the scope and the precision of his observations and to facilitate data recall and correlation. Micromethods will be perfected to the extent that a miniscular amount of material from a patient can be analyzed for many determinations.

To the seriously interested scientist, pathology offers an opportunity unequaled by any other specialty to study all aspects of disease. In pathology an investigator has direct access to the special knowledge and skill of other branches of biology and medicine for application to basic or applied research. In pathology a physician has an unexcelled opportunity to teach the causes, the processes and the effects of disease to his medical colleagues, residents, interns, medical students, technicians, nurses and others. In pathology a scientist has a golden opportunity to serve society and the medical profession and to derive boundless inner satisfaction as a leader, practitioner, investigator and teacher in the diagnosis, the prevention and the understanding of human ills.

BIBLIOGRAPHY AND REFERENCES

1. Wartman, W. B.: Training of pathologists *in* Yearbook of Pathology and Clinical Pathology, pp. 7-12, Chicago, Yearbook Medical Publishers, 1961-62.

2. Long, E. R.: A History of American Pathology, Springfield, Ill., Thomas, 1962.

3. Directory of Approved Internships and Residencies. Supplement to J.A.M.A. *182*, No. 7, 336 pp., 1962. (Copies available on request to Council on Medical Education and Hospitals, American Medical Association, 535 North Dearborn Street, Chicago 10, Ill.)

4. Beerman, H., and Pillsbury, D.: Dermatopathology as a field of research, Lab. Invest. *6*:389-411, 1957.

5. McManus, J. F. A.: The trend toward a molecular pathology, Lab. Invest. *6*:289-292, 1957.

6. A Career in Medical Science; Pathology. Intersociety Committee for Research Potential in Pathology. (A 33-page illustrated brochure; copies available upon request to Dr. T. D. Kinney, Secretary-Treasurer of the Intersociety Committee for Research Potential in Pathology, Inc., Duke University Medical Center, Durham, N. C.)

7. Hass, G.: The hospital pathologist—practitioner, educator or scientist?, Lab. Invest. *6*:389-411, 1957.

8. Symposium on increasing the research potential in pathology, Lab. Invest. *3*:378-450, 1954.

9. American Society of Clinical Pathologists, 445 North Lake Shore Drive, Chicago 11, Ill.

10. College of American Pathologists, Prudential Plaza, Chicago 1, Ill.

LUTHER L. TERRY, M.D.

Surgeon General, U. S. Public Health Service

22

The Physician in the Federal Government

No group of the many members of the medical profession in this country can feel a greater sense of personal satisfaction than the group which serves the health programs of the Federal Government. Bound by the Hippocratic oath, which pledges them to "lend their lives and practice their art with uprightness and honor," these men and women are active participants in world-wide efforts to improve human health and to make life better and longer for all people.

The opportunities offered are varied and unique. In hospitals operated by the Public Health Service, the Army, the Navy, the Air Force and the Veterans Administration, a physician has every chance to practice clinical medicine. In the Air Force he can become a flight surgeon; in the Navy, a submarine medical officer. If he is interested in research, all services offer many opportunities in this field. The National Institutes of Health, a part of the Public Health Service, are considered the foremost research center in the world. Foreign assignments await those in the military services and, in some cases, those in the Commissioned Corps of the Public Health Service, a quasimilitary service. Here the physician may find himself caring for his fellow Americans abroad or for peoples of other countries. He may make an unusual contribution to the health of an underdeveloped country, or he may act as a medical adviser to a foreign government.

The opportunities offered are stimulating and broadening. A physician working within the government framework can serve the health of the family, the community and the nation— on the broadest possible basis. If he is interested, he can see things from a national or state or community vantage point. He has an excellent chance, if he so chooses, to exercise latent administrative skills. The physician with ability for leadership never will want for opportunities in government service.

Indeed, because of the latitude of the medical responsibilities of the Federal Government, the opportunities of the physician for professional growth and personal satisfaction in administration, practice, teaching and research are unparalleled.

FEDERAL HEALTH FUNCTIONS

As an agency of the Department of Health, Education and Welfare, the Public Health Service is the principal health agency of the Federal Government. It has a definite responsibility in the broad fields of health, research and training; medical care for legally designated beneficiaries; and public health practices, including the development of resources, facilities and technics. It is responsible also for certain direct services, such as interstate and foreign quarantine, and for working with other countries on matters of international health.

Many other government agencies have health functions that are secondary or supplementary to their main mission. Thus the Departments of the Army, the Navy and the Air Force, the Veterans Administration and the Department of Justice administer medical services for military personnel and their dependents, veterans and Federal prisons, respectively. The Department of State operates a small medical program for Foreign Service personnel on duty outside the United States and provides physical examinations for the attaché program of the Department of Agriculture.

PUBLIC HEALTH SERVICE

There are numerous opportunities for physicians in the Public Health Service in the fields of clinical and preventive medicine, public health and research.

The Service is working currently in broad areas of hospital care, chronic diseases and aging, and community and environmental health. Research and control programs concern cancer, heart disease, arthritis and metabolic diseases, mental illness, allergy and infectious diseases, neurologic diseases and blindness, water supply and pollution control, accident prevention, radiologic health and air pollution.

Opportunities for clinical practice, training and research prevail in the 15 U. S. Public Health Service hospitals located throughout the country. These hospitals range in size up to 1,050 beds and provide care and treatment for American merchant seamen, officers and enlisted men of the U. S. Coast Guard and their dependents, Federal employees injured at work, officers and crew members of the Coast and Geodetic Survey.

Twelve of these provide general medical and surgical care. Two—one at Lexington, Ky., and the other at Fort Worth, Tex.—treat narcotic addiction and other neuropsychiatric disorders. The combination hospital and community at Carville, La., is the national leprosarium.

More than 50 other hospitals are operated for the care and the treatment of American Indians and Alaskan natives. Opportunities for training, teaching and research exist at all levels.

PHS provides medical, surgical, psychiatric and dental services for nearly 25,000 prisoners in 30 Federal institutions located in 21 states. All of the hospitals in the larger institutions and many of those in the smaller institutions are fully accredited by the AMA Joint Commission on Accreditation of Hospitals. These institutions of the Bureau of Prisons provide a variety of cases.

Many of the PHS medical officers are engaged in research.

The principal research center of the Service is the National Institutes of Health at Bethesda, Md., which conducts laboratory and clinical investigations on the major diseases of mankind. Research is under way also at various facilities throughout the country on environmental health problems, including radiologic health. The Communicable Disease Center in Atlanta, Ga., where the emphasis is on epidemiology and control, is a national resource in the fight against communicable disease. The NIH Middle America Research Unit in the Panama Canal Zone concentrates on studies of anthropod-borne viruses and other health problems best observed in the tropics. The Arctic Health Research Center in Anchorage, Alaska, is the headquarters for investigations of the effects of low temperature and the Arctic environment on life and health.

To prevent contagious diseases from entering the country, PHS medical officers keep vigil at 20 major seaports and land border ports in the United States and insular possessions. They examine visa applicants and serve as technical advisers to consular officials at major United States consulates in foreign countries. Similarly, they perform quarantine inspection and medical examinations of Mexican laborers at border reception centers in California, Arizona and Texas.

The Public Health Service also details professional personnel to the medical programs of other Federal agencies. These are the Federal Employee Health Program, the U. S. Coast Guard and the Coast and Geodetic Survey, the Peace Corps, and the Bureau of Employees' Compensation of the U. S. Department of Labor.

Almost all the PHS physicians are members of the Service's Commissioned Corps, a career officer organization established in 1873. While the Corps was formed to provide a mobile force of physicians who would serve where assigned, today it includes dentists, sanitary engineers, nurses, scientists, social workers and other categories of professional personnel.

The Commissioned Corps consists of a Regular Corps of career Officers—limited in size by law—and a Reserve Corps that augments the Regular Corps to the extent program needs require and funds permit. Rank and salaries are comparable with those in the Armed Forces, and PHS officers are expected to serve wherever the needs of the Service take them. In addition to base pay, they receive a rental and subsistence allowance. Two years of active duty in the Corps satisfies selective service obligation.

There are several ways to enter the Corps:

1. Through the Commissioned Officer Student Training and Extern Program (COSTEP), available to second- and third-year medical students who apply for Reserve commissions and active duty during vacation periods.

2. Through the medical intern program in PHS hospitals affiliated with major teaching centers. Interns hold Reserve commissions equivalent to that of Navy Lieutenants or Army Captains.

3. As a general duty medical officer in the grade of Senior Assistant Surgeon, following one year's internship either at a PHS hospital or at an approved hospital outside the Service.

4. As a clinical resident in training at a PHS hospital or the Clinical Center of the National Institutes of Health; or as a public health resident on assignment to a state health department.

The Service, with the authorization of the Selective Service System, conducts the Commissioned Officer Residency Deferment (CORD) Program. Draft-eligible physicians are commissioned in the Inactive Reserve Corps and deferred while completing residency training in civilian hospitals. These physicians are committed to serve their Selective Service time with the Public Health Service and are called to active duty immediately after the completion of residency training. No additional obligatory military service under the Draft Act is required.

DEPARTMENT OF THE ARMY

The Army Medical Service has five broad objectives: the practice of medicine, field medicine or combat readiness, medical education and training, medical research and development, and medical administration and management.

To further these objectives this Service has concentrated its major efforts in two basic areas of interest: (1) to render the highest caliber of medical care possible to its beneficiaries by using the most highly qualified physicians and the most modern and advanced drugs and equipment; and (2) constant research and development to discover the cause of disease, to develop preventives or curatives and to develop new or better life-saving surgical materials. In addition, the Army Medical Service endeavors to develop, field test and adopt new medical equipment which will increase the mobility and the efficiency of field medical units and thus fulfill its age-old mandate—to conserve the fighting strength of the Army.

Most physicians entering active duty with the Army attend the Army Medical Service Officer Orientation Course. Then as general-duty medical officers they may be assigned directly to duty or apply for specialized training. In the former instance they are assigned within the continental United States or overseas to field units, dispensaries or hospitals.

Those who wish to specialize may apply for training in one of the clinical specialties, preventive medicine, aviation medicine or other fields. Thus the Army physician may find himself in duty assignments of increasing responsibility, or he may be studying the health problems and disease hazards that exist wherever American troops are stationed or are likely to serve, or he may be fulfilling the demand for intensified medical activity in the field of aviation.

The Army Medical Service recognizes that rapid technologic advances are characteristic of both the medical and the military professions. Therefore, it feels that research and developments in clinical medicine, basic science, preventive medicine, nuclear medicine and combat development activities must be evaluated and adapted for maximum benefit to its mission.

Officers selected for this duty usually have prior training

in clinical, preventive or aviation medicine and have demonstrated an interest in and an aptitude for research. They attend the Military Medicine and Allied Science Course and are then assigned to various research installations.

Those having an interest in nuclear training may receive further training in this field. By virtue of this training they are then equipped to plan, direct and supervise medical aspects of operations involving nuclear weapons, radioactive materials and radiation-producing equipment. They also serve as military staff advisers in the field of nuclear energy.

There is a continuing need for the understanding and the utilization of management principles and technics used throughout the Medical Service. Key positions in this area are filled by Medical Corps officers. Although many officers will serve primarily in this field, others serve only one tour and then re-enter their primary or another career field.

The Army offers a number of programs for medical students and graduates. They are:

1. The Army Residency program, which has established over 500 residencies in 25 specialties and subspecialties in Army teaching hospitals. Training in civilian hospitals is authorized only when the specialty needs of the Army cannot be met by training in these Army hospitals.

2. The Army Internship program, which provides essential experience in the field of medicine. The program includes surgery, medicine, pediatrics, obstetrics and gynecology, followed by elective assignments in such fields as ophthalmology, otolaryngology, radiology, psychiatry and neurology, and physical medicine.

3. The Army Senior Medical Student program, which provides a limited number of appointments in the Army Reserve to seniors in medical schools in the United States and Puerto Rico. These students are called to active duty at the beginning of their senior year and remain until graduation.

4. The Clinical Clerkship Training program, which provides the rising junior or senior medical student with an

opportunity to serve for not more than 60 days in one of the major teaching hospitals of the Army, either as a lieutenant in a Reserve component or in civil service status.

DEPARTMENT OF THE NAVY

The medical officer in the Navy is provided every opportunity to practice clinical and preventive medicine in the 25 U. S. Naval hospitals located throughout the United States and outside its continental limits.

A number of these are general hospitals serving active duty and retired naval personnel and their dependents, but special treatment facilities are available at others. A special feature of one is a Radiation Exposure Evaluation Laboratory, while several others have special facilities for open-heart surgery, cardiac catheterization, vascular surgery, thoracic surgery and neurosurgery. Still another specializes in plastic surgery, deep x-ray, radium, oncology and cardiopulmonary function.

While the Naval submarine medical program is a small one, it offers career advancement and personal enrichment. Submarine medicine has two general programs, the conventional submarine program and the nuclear submarine program.

The majority of physicians in the former program serve as squadron medical officers on the staffs of submarine squadron commanders. Here the medical officer has over-all responsibility for some 2,000 officers and men. The squadron includes a submarine tender, containing a 34-bed hospital, and a diving ship. The medical officer is responsible for medical supervision of squadron deep-sea diving operations and care of the divers.

The nuclear submarine program is the newest and one of the most interesting parts of the Navy. It carries with it unique medical problems. A medical officer is assigned to a new nuclear submarine, and he remains as a crew member for a period of 6 to 12 months.

Research in submarine medicine is available for those interested in research and teaching assignments. Of great importance are the research programs in respiratory physiology and in assessment of personnel for submarine duty.

The Naval flight surgeon performs a vital service for his country by aiding in the selection of top-quality personnel who must carry out complex mental tasks in hazardous environments. His job does not end there. He is responsible also for maintaining that personnel at maximum effectiveness.

The flight surgeon may combine his aviation medicine with a clinical specialty, such as ophthalmology, medicine, surgery otorhinolaryngology, psychiatry and others. Certification in pathology, in addition to aviation, is another example of a long-range career pattern for flight surgeons.

The Navy provides a wide variety of research opportunities for medical officers interested in this field. In addition to aviation and submarine medicine, laboratory research is conducted in clinical specialties, amphibious and field medicine, tropical and exotic diseases, and the medical aspects of nuclear, biologic and chemical warfare defense. These 15 research laboratories are located throughout the world.

The Navy offers:

1. Approved residency training in every major specialty and subspecialty of medicine and surgery in selected U. S. Naval hospitals, and, depending on the needs of the service, in a number of civilian medical schools and centers throughout the country.

2. One hundred and seventy-six rotating internships each year, through the National Intern Matching Program, Inc. This training is provided in 13 Naval hospitals, selected for their excellent facilities and for the available clinical material. Eight of the hospitals also provide residency training and are located in areas in or near civilian teaching centers. Here the intern training is similar to that in university training.

3. The Ensign, Probationary (Medical) Program, which provides that a medical student may join the Naval Reserve with the rank of Ensign and continue his education in an accredited medical school. This provision assures both defer-

ment from active duty until graduation and that the period of active duty will be with the Navy's Medical Department.

UNITED STATES AIR FORCE

The Medical Corps offers career opportunities in two distinct areas, both important in providing adequate medical care for the Air Force, clinical medicine and aerospace medicine.

Clinical medicine includes direct medical care and treatment in clinics, dispensaries and hospitals.

Aerospace medicine includes but is not limited to medical evaluation of and periodic re-evaluation of flying personnel; unit medical care; aerospace medical research and development; aerospace medical teaching; medical aspects of flying safety, rescue and survival; and aeromedical evacuation.

Research may be performed in either clinical medicine or aerospace medicine. The former concerns the study and treatment of specific diseases, including the evaluation of drugs and methods, while the latter deals chiefly with research in the areas of human-factor requirements in aerospace medicine and the development of equipment to help man meet these requirements.

The Air Force is engaged currently in a hospital construction program that eventually will comprise 241 new medical and dental facilities both in the United States and overseas.

There are now over 130 hospitals, which range in bed capacity from 25 to 1,000 beds. They run the geographic gamut from Alaska to Tripoli to the Azores. One of the features of these hospitals is that each is adapted to the prevailing temperature in its particular climate.

The Air Force has planned medical support for its installations based on the needs of the installation itself. The smaller bases are staffed with general practitioners and physicians in the broader medical specialties, while the larger bases have all the medical specialties plus emphasis on a preventive medical program allied with the clinical program.

The outstanding medical specialty center in Europe is a

350-bed hospital at Wiesbaden, Germany. Here care is available in internal medicine, general surgery, obstetrics-gynecology, cardiopulmonary diseases, gastroenterology, contagious diseases, orthopedic surgery, thoracic surgery, dermatology, pediatrics, urology, otolaryngology, ophthalmology, neurosurgery, anesthesiology and psychiatry. In addition, the hospital includes complete laboratory, pharmacy and radiologic services, as well as a modern dental service.

The Air Force Flight Surgeon is a graduate of the School of Aerospace Medicine, part of the new Aerospace Medical Center in Texas. He has received a primary course of 350 hours in physiology, biometrics, biophysics, aviation psychology, preventive and space medicine and related sciences. After a year of duty he may apply for admission to the Aviation Medicine Specialty Training Program.

The first phase of this training is a graduate course in preventive medicine at a recognized civilian university. For this a degree of Master of Public Health—or its equivalent—is awarded. In the second phase wide use is made of clinical practice. The student learns technics that conserve the health and the efficiency of flying personnel. He takes also eight weeks of flight indoctrination to gain actual experience of the medical conditions and problems of flight. The third phase is a one-year residency. This enables the physician to gain additional experience and skill in preventive medicine and other closely related aviation medicine specialties.

The Air Force offers:

1. Residencies in general practice or in specialties in military and civilian hospitals. The programs in the former last for 2 years and generally provide for 1 year of training in medicine and 1 year in surgery. In the latter the Air Force will sponsor formal training only for the minimum period of time required by the specific specialty board.

2. A Civilian Intern Program that may commission current medical school graduates for assignment to the civilian hospitals in which they have obtained approved internships.

3. A Military Intern Program, in which graduates of medical schools are selected on a competitive basis each year to receive intern training as Air Force officers in military teaching hospitals.

4. A Student Program, whereby selected students are placed on extended active duty that lasts through the date of formal graduation. During the senior year they must apply for training in either the Military or Civilian Intern Program.

VETERANS ADMINISTRATION

The Medical Care Program of the Veterans Administration is one of the largest of its kind in the Federal Government. It comprises 125,000 hospital beds, 114,000 hospital patients and 7,878 physicians. Its operational control includes 10 per cent of the hospital beds and 7 per cent of the physicians in the nation.

In addition to its 120 general medical and surgical hospitals, the Veterans Administration operates 39 hospitals designated for neuropsychiatric patients and 11 for patients with tuberculosis or chronic chest diseases.

The Veterans Administration offers the physician who has completed his internship a progressive medical program in a professional environment, extensive opportunity for research, a graduate program of medical education and completely modern research, surgical, diagnostic and auxiliary medical equipment.

DEPARTMENT OF STATE

In addition to care for its own employees overseas, the Department of State supervises medical services for the Agency for International Development (AID) and the United States Information Agency (USIA) employees overseas. Fifteen physicians and 35 nurses are stationed abroad. In Washington several staff physicians serve in administrative capacities, and a number of part-time physicians work on a contract basis.

CIVIL SERVICE COMMISSION

Currently, through the Civil Service Commission over 1,000 medical officers are employed in the Federal Government. Some of these hold civilian jobs in the agencies just described, and others are employed by the Atomic Energy Commission, the National Aeronautics and Space Administration, the Food and Drug Administration and the Children's Bureau.

The physician in Government—whatever his field, wherever his assignment—can feel a great sense of accomplishment, a great sense of challenge. He may find a demanding career, but it is sure to be a rewarding one. This career could take him to the depths of the ocean or into space, or it could bring him fame in the world of research. More important than that, he will be an integral part of efforts aimed at a larger goal. He will be one of many who are making unselfish and humanitarian contributions to the quest for better health for all people throughout the world.

WILLIAM B. BEAN, M.D.

*Professor of Medicine and Head of the Department of
Internal Medicine at the University of Iowa*

23

Caritas Medici

What may be said of the functions, the duties and the obligations of the physician as a man of good will and as a citizen? The answer does not call for cant, for polished platitudes and the glittering words of so many formal talks or graduation addresses. One must resist the pleasure of that species of pomposity that masquerades as wisdom—a peculiar occupational hazard of all doctors—and the false sophistication of professors whose very title connotes a risk of pedantry and sophistry.

Let him remember in all his dealings with those who come to him for help that the patient is *sick,* or believes himself to be. Often he cares little or nothing about the scientific diagnosis or even the name of his trouble. He needs help, assurance, reassurance and relief from pain or distress. The well-trained physician wants to find out the nature of the trouble, remove it, diminish it, palliate it or if these cannot be done, to help the patient to accept it. Some patients seek help with diseases for which there is no radical corrective therapy.

In order to succeed in one's mission one must teach the patient how to be an active partner in the program for his own salvation. Patients do not gladly accept a primary role in regaining health. They want the easy way—something produced by the mystery of medicine, or a miracle drug. They want the evil cut out. Only rarely will they do their part without clear explanation and instruction and, of course, not always even then. A strange perverseness in human nature may frustrate one's best and most thoughtful efforts. It is important to realize that in the social transaction that is the basis of the practice of medicine the patient and the physician may begin at odds. In order that the patient who is looking for comfort and relief does not become annoyed or frustrated by the physician's concentration on diagnosis, he must be encouraged to talk. He must also be listened to. Give him full and undivided attention. Part of the vast neurosis of contemporary life resides in the inability to attend. Only the very best physicians ever become masters of attending completely without intruding.

But all of us can become sympathetic listeners. In this we practice good therapy. Do not lose the patient's confidence by sending him away for a battery of tests before telling him not only where and when but something of what and why. It is not necessary for a physician to have had an illness to understand something about that illness, but it does deepen his perception. Imagination helps. If one has been on the receiving end of gastric analyses, catheterizations, venipunctures, barium enemas and the like, one has a new insight into the vast difference between giving and receiving. One may see more deeply into the reactions to be expected of a sick, frightened, bewildered patient to whom the physician, at least in the beginning, is a stranger before becoming a guide and friend.

In short, one must escape from the protracted adolescence of contemporary man whose hunger for pleasure and happiness often expresses itself in boorishness, vulgarity and petty meanness. This is always distressing but can be disastrous in a physician. All too often a doctor and a nurse, an orderly or someone else caring for the sick may exhibit peevishness, meanness, a quick temper, inattention or just some trifling lack of consideration that nullifies the efforts of brilliant science and technical virtuosity. For this disorder the simplest cure in the world is to put oneself in the place of one's patient.

As with most admonitions this is easy to say but hard to do.

It may seem strange that much of the misunderstanding in the world today inheres in the casual acceptance of a superficial conception of words and language. Too many physicians in their rush to acquire preprofessional technics and certainly in the course of their undergraduate training in medical school neglected the vital mastery of their native tongue. Comprehension of ideas depends on words and language. As the medium of learning, words are the framework upon which special training is built and held together. They determine the course of one's day-by-day dealing with patients and with the world. A strange but rather pervasive hostility to excellence has led many people in modern times to fear culture as though it were a perversion of normal behavior. No one can do an effective job in a profession unless he sweeps aside the childish notion that culture correlates with effeminacy. It is never too late for those who have neglected this essential aspect of existence to make a start by gaining some familiarity with the thoughts, the words and the deeds of the finest and greatest members of the human race throughout all the ages. Substantial ground can be gained by the habit of regular daily reading of the classics, history, English—indeed, any of the world's great literatures. This requires determination and persistence. If one achieves a thorough command of language based on an understanding of its purpose and of history, he will avoid the prevailing sin of obscurity and confusion of ideas and the failure to perceive and act upon the profound difference between fact and fancy.

Man alone can comprehend time and apply a tenuous check rein to it by profiting from the cumulative experience of the past. But this he may not do unless he understands completely the subtle but essential distinction between words, ideas and things. Without this he can never make any sense out of history and he must remember the all-encompassing warning of Santayana that "those who cannot remember the past are condemned to repeat it."

As one deals with patients he must realize that in the strict sense every patient is a "test subject," and every operation, treatment, regimen or program is an "experiment"; but do not use the word experiment in the hearing of patients and never mention human guinea pigs. Words are subtle, slippery, changing chameleons. They leave our lips with what we think is a clear intent, but they may be heard with different implications and meanings. Misunderstood or dislodged from their proper context they may be frightening; or they may be clutched at as straws of false hope. They should not be inadvertent sources of anguish as when a casual word, overheard, is interpreted as a sentence of death or invalidism. The traditional long words of the physician are of great annoyance to the patient, whether sophisticated or unsophisticated. It makes a further and unnecessary barrier between them. A good system is to use words that an intelligent child can understand, without at the same time talking down to the patient. Avoid unfamiliar technical terms. Most patients can take a term such as electrocardiogram in stride but may be bewildered by dyspnea or polychondritis.

An example of the unfortunate depersonalization of medicine, a source of some anguish and so much outspoken hostility to physicians, is the use of those old zoologic labels, male and female. It is just as accurate and easier to say man or woman, boy or girl. This avoids the implication that the patient is a specimen or the subject of an experiment. And even more important, it removes the strong, but usually unmeant implication of intellectual or social superiority. We do not refer to our mother as a charming, 50-, 60- or 70-year-old white female. Such crude usage, usually passed over without a thought, is another manifestation of the dehumanization of medicine that patients resent, though in their quiet acceptance they may say little about it.

An equally unpleasant custom is the reference to patients as cases, particularly within their hearing. A case means an example, an item or an element of data. A case cannot have a lesion, though there may be many cases of a particular lesion. Perhaps unintended insults to patients persist because we

never quite shake off the physician-cadaver relation that constituted our introduction into medical school. Probably much
of the public's increasing hostility to "doctors" stems from the
patient's objection to being relegated to the role of an inani-
mate item or statistic. Patients naturally resent being thought
of as physical vehicles (and a great nuisance at that) for beguil-
ing lesions or enchanting processes.

Another occupational hazard of the physician, especially
the young one, is the tendency to use a long word, sometimes
erroneously, where a short one, easier to use and remember,
often gives a clearer and more precise meaning. One might
list a hundred words commonly misused, but a few examples
will suffice. When we mean "lesion" we say "pathology,"
though when admiring the starry heavens few of us say "how
fine the astronomy," or when commenting on a charming
flower garden we do not find it necessary to say "how delightful the horticulture." The patient may properly be on a bed
or on a bedpan, but not on digitalis or on a high fat diet,
unless he has fallen into the soup. Avoidance of long words
is not an absolute law but a good one to observe in our talks
with patients. A little practice will enable us to make the
appropriate translation from the vernacular or simple idio-
matic English into concepts of pathophysiology that will enable us to understand some of the mechanisms of illness.
Then we have to make a translation back into terms that will
enable the patient to understand our meaning and become
our colleague in the proper management of his care and, as
often as possible, his cure.

It may seem distressing to have to remind physicians about
good manners that should be axiomatic. But physicians young
and old have not escaped the corroding blight of modern
times and modern education—the lack of thoughtfulness and
consideration for others. As an example of this, the casual
term "LMD" or local medical doctor is used too often with
the implication that those in other institutions or other places
are inadequate or incompetent. Absent colleagues and referring physicians should be respected. Too many disturbed or

unscrupulous persons today are ready to bring suit for non-existent damages because of some casually dropped remark or gesture. The look of surprise, the hint of negligence or stupidity may plant the seed of a law suit, and even if it has no such result it is a needless and hostile act. If one resorts to the simple expedient of acting as if the referring physician were in the room nothing is likely to be said or listened to that would imply stupidity or point to a scapegoat. This is not the same as hiding malpractice or an error committed to the patient's detriment. Since patients have a wonderful talent for misunderstanding, for gossip or for sheer invention, one should get the facts before judging and certainly before blaming.

We are all too busy. The tensions of facing problems and making decisions on which life and death hinge, which physicians must face every day, easily result in short tempers, fatigue, or even exhaustion. Courtesy must be remembered no matter how much it costs in time and thoughtfulness. A place where this is especially apt to be deficient is in requesting consultations. We should keep in mind that childish eruptions of temper often mean some fault on the part of the donor rather than on that of the recipient of the outburst. Remember the formal graces of consultation of yesteryear, not to duplicate a hollow ritual but to recognize that in such circumstances courtesy and manners were evolved to make difficult situations easier for physician, consultant, the family itself and, not least, the patient. The request for consultation should be made personally or reviewed by the physician if his secretary fills out the paper. It should include the nature of the problem, the reason for the consultation, what is desired in specific terms (not "have 'dermatology' see him") and the degree of urgency. Sending records may be helpful, but they should never be available as casual reading material for the patient. If a particular physician is needed he should be called personally and not by shouting down the hall. The request for laboratory tests is essentially a request for consultation, although routine request forms are valuable as labor-saving devices. We should remember that the essence of the relation is that of colleagues working together.

When troubles arise in our dealings with our colleagues or with patients—and in the nature of things troubles do arise—one should get to the heart of the matter immediately by getting specific facts. Go at once to the person or persons concerned. Never wait until tomorrow. Don't sulk. Don't brood. Perhaps it is your fault. It may be the fault of the system, the times or the wonderfully fallible nature of man. But do not let it erode your spirit or corrode your good will and produce unnecessary hurt or turn into an enemy one who might be a friend. The tattletale and the gossip have no place in medicine. In our time with its signs of mounting tension and increasing vocal hostility toward the medical profession, it is well to remember that something may be wrong with some of the members of that profession. Certainly there is a distorted mental image of the physician. One of the major duties of physicians today is to correct this bad public impression of themselves by improving their relations with patients and by applying the proper countercurrent of example and precept. The reasons for complaint must be reduced to the barest minimum so that the physician, the student of medicine and the whole company of hospital people not only avoid evil but avoid the appearance of evil. We must give no offense by not being offensive. It is by cultivating the proper attitudes and ideals rather than imposing a set of rules that we do our best work and create the most favorable impression. Fortunately, the proper goals of both patient and physician are served simultaneously. If we do our best our inevitable failures will be tolerable, but even more important, they will become infrequent.

Since no one is perfect, despite the best intentions, we may feel a little self-conscious in delivering admonitions concerning integrity and intellectual honesty. Everyone is well aware that a person is ultimately destroyed if he habitually departs from honesty. But especially in professions that depend on personal relations there is no substitute for absolute integrity. In certain educational institutions students are lined up in a hostile camp on one side, the teachers and the instructors on the other, and a contest is waged. The student wants to see what one can get away with. Dishonesty is corrosive. No method of internal segregation or quarantine can allow one to be honest in all save one or a few areas. In medicine those infected with dishonesty may survive for a time but sooner or later the blight will damage others and so destroy them. At all times one's dealings with patients, with colleagues and with friends should be characterized by complete honesty.

Many essays have dealt with various aspects of what a physician should and should not tell patients. It should be axiomatic that though one does not have to say all he knows or all he thinks he knows, any system that condones evasiveness, the half truth or the out-and-out lie will result in more trouble than good. Telling the truth does not mean the compulsive spouting forth of bad news in bleak and unadorned terms. A single truth may be conveyed in many ways. For instance, in a clinical disorder that has a mortality rate of approximately 25 per cent I like to emphasize to the patient that three fourths of all people with such trouble get well, while at the same time a responsible member of the family is informed that a quarter of the patients die. Here the same fact is presented with a different emphasis, though the truth contained in the two statements will be perceived well enough by all concerned. No law can hold good for all patients and all conditions. Here simple humanity must guide us, for every patient and every phase of disease requires individual consideration and action. If we strive for honesty with humility we may achieve wisdom in our deeds. In times when a patient is profoundly ill, or death is approaching, we do well to hold fast to William Jenner's triad of essential qualities for the medical man: "He must be honest, he must be dogmatic and he must be kind."

I will try to summarize these remarks by reverting to a theme I have expounded elsewhere in a talk to undergraduate medical students. I defined the physician's essential quality as "*Caritas Medici*," using the Latin words because they not only defined the mores of the physician of good will but embodied them in a rich expression with the freshness of the early morning dew still on it. The expression "bedside manner," now much abused, captures some of the meaning. *Caritas,* through vagrant changes, gives us charity and care and carries implications of love and tenderness and dearness —of "loving kindness." But *caritas medici,* a physician's *caritas,* means much more. It is that vigilant and humane insight and care, compact of wisdom and spirit, which the doctor owes his patient, be it for sympathy or discipline. This concept Francis Peabody epitomized beautifully for us once and for all in his statement that "The secret of the care of the patient is in caring for the patient."

I conclude with two more paragraphs from the same address: " 'Go calmly amid the daily hurly-burly.' Remember the peace there is in silence. Be on good terms with people. Speak your truth quietly and convincingly but listen to others; they have their side to tell. Avoid loudness and aggression. Comparisons are to no purpose for there are always greater and smaller persons than yourself. Enjoy your plans as well as your achievements. Keep a vital interest in your own professional life and progress, a real possession in the changing fortunes of time. Do not let dishonesty blind you to the fact that virtue exists. Be true, be yourself, and be true to yourself. Do not feign love nor simulate affection. Neither be ironic about love. In the face of all disillusionment and disenchantment, it is as perennial as the grass. Grow old gracefully, surrendering at appropriate times the things of youth. Do not borrow trouble with dark imaginings. Be gentle. You are a child of the universe no less than the stars and the trees, and whether you see it or not, no doubt the universe is unfolding as it should. Be at peace with God, whatever you conceive him to be. In the noisy confusion of life be at peace with your soul."

"Finally, I end with a quotation from Tennyson's *Idylls of the King,* which I think might be as profitable reading for many of us as the latest installment in the mystery of the isotope. I quote:

> "For manners are not idle, but the fruit
>   Of loyal nature and of noble mind."